A 48-WEEK HOLISTIC
DEVOTIONAL

Health &
Discipleship

ADAM WOOD

Cover Design by Yasir Nadeem

Book Design by HMDPUBLISHING

Adam Wood

(217) 260-7635

hello@therevwood.com

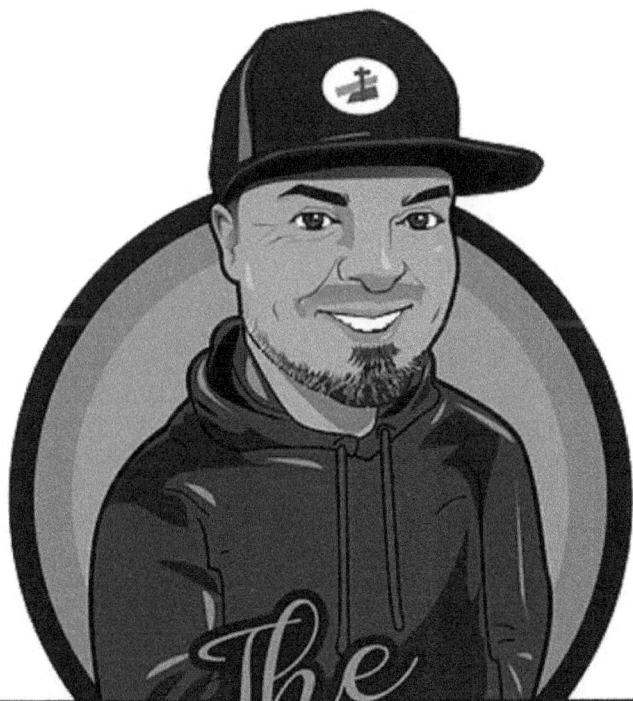

The REV WOOD

.com

CONTENTS

INTRODUCTION

WHAT IS HOLISTIC HEALTH?

Holistic health in the context of the Christian life encompasses the integration of spiritual, physical, mental, and financial well-being, all of which are interconnected and essential components of a balanced and thriving life. Embracing holistic health as a Christian involves nurturing and caring for each aspect of our being, recognizing that God desires wholeness and flourishing in every area of our lives.

Spiritual Health:

- Spiritual health is foundational to holistic well-being for Christians, as it involves cultivating a deep and intimate relationship with God through faith in Jesus Christ. This includes regular spiritual practices such as prayer, Bible study, worship, and fellowship with other believers. Spiritual health also involves aligning our lives with God's will, seeking His guidance and direction, and living out our faith in love and obedience.

Physical Health:

- Physical health encompasses caring for our bodies as temples of the Holy Spirit (1 Corinthians 6:19-20). This involves maintaining a balanced diet, engaging in regular exercise, getting adequate rest, and avoiding harmful habits such as substance abuse. As stewards of our bodies, Christians are called to honor God by prioritizing self-care and pursuing optimal physical health.

Mental Health:

- Mental health involves nurturing our minds and emotional well-being. This includes managing stress, cultivating positive thought patterns, seeking support when needed, and practicing self-care activities that promote mental resilience and emotional balance. Christians are encouraged to renew their minds with God's Word (Romans 12:2) and to cast their cares upon Him (1 Peter 5:7), trusting in His provision and comfort during times of difficulty.

Financial Health:

- Financial health encompasses stewardship of the resources God has entrusted to us, including finances, possessions, and material resources. This involves living within our means, avoiding debt, practicing generosity, and using our resources to advance God's Kingdom purposes. Christians are called to seek first God's Kingdom and trust in His provision for their needs (Matthew 6:33), recognizing that true wealth is found in relationship with Him rather than in material possessions.

In summary, holistic health in the Christian life involves nurturing and caring for our spiritual, physical, mental, and financial well-being, recognizing that each aspect is interconnected and essential to experiencing abundant life in Christ. By prioritizing holistic health, Christians can honor God with their whole selves and fulfill their God-given purpose to love and serve others in His name.

OVERVIEW OF DEVOTIONAL STRUCTURE

Welcome to this 48-week devotional journey on holistic health! This guided section is designed to help you make the most of your experience as you delve into the principles of spiritual, physical, mental, and financial well-being according to God's Word. Each week, you will explore a different aspect of holistic health through Scripture readings, reflections, prayers, and practical exercises.

GETTING STARTED

- Set aside dedicated time: Choose a consistent time each day or week to engage with the devotional. Whether it's in the morning, during lunch breaks, or before bedtime, establish a routine that works for you.

- Create a sacred space: Find a quiet and comfortable environment where you can focus on your devotional time without distractions. Consider lighting a candle, playing soft music, or surrounding yourself with inspiring imagery to enhance your experience.

- Open your heart: Approach each devotional session with an open heart and mind, ready to receive the insights and truths that God has in store for you. Pray for guidance as you embark on this journey of spiritual growth and transformation.

NAVIGATING THE DEVOTIONAL

- Follow the weekly structure: Each week of the devotional is dedicated to a specific theme related to holistic health, such as spiritual renewal, physical wellness, emotional resilience, or financial stewardship. If you miss a week here and there, that's fine. We've designed this with 48 weeks instead of 52 weeks so that you have a buffer.

- Engage with Scripture: Dive into the selected Bible passages provided for each week's theme. Reflect on the verses, meditate on their meaning, and consider how they apply to your life. Don't shy away from reading the surrounding Scripture as well, so you fully understand the context.

- Reflect and journal: Take time to ponder the discussion questions and prompts provided in the devotional. Journal your thoughts, insights, and prayers as you process the Scripture readings and apply them to your own journey toward holistic health.

- Pray and seek guidance: Spend time in prayer, seeking God's wisdom, guidance, and strength as you explore the principles of holistic health. Offer your concerns, hopes, and desires to God, and ask Him to empower you to live out His truth in every area of your life.

- Take action: Apply what you've learned from each week's devotional to your daily life. Implement practical steps and habits that align with God's principles for holistic health, whether it's practicing self-care, nurturing relationships, stewarding your finances, or deepening your spiritual walk.

- Connect with others: Consider participating in a small group or community where you can discuss the devotional content, share insights, and encourage one another on your journey toward holistic health. Accountability and support from fellow believers can enrich your experience and foster spiritual growth.

CONCLUSION

As you embark on this 48-week devotional journey on holistic health, may you be blessed with spiritual insights, renewed strength, and transformative growth. May God's Word illuminate your path, His Spirit guide your steps, and His presence sustain you through every season of life. May you experience the fullness of His abundant life as you pursue holistic health in body, mind, and spirit. Amen.

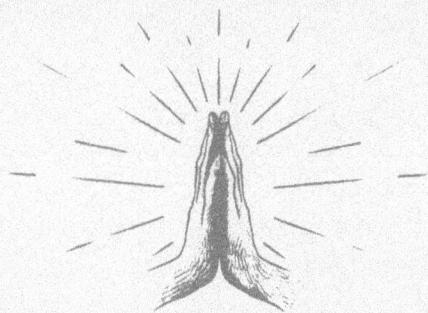

Spiritual Health

WEEK 1:

RELATIONSHIP WITH GOD

JAMES 4:8 (NIV)

"Come near to God and he will come near to you. Wash your hands, you sinners, and purify your hearts, you double-minded."

DEVOTION

The pursuit of a deep and intimate relationship with God is at the core of our Christian journey. James, in his letter, offers a profound invitation and instruction regarding our relationship with God. He urges us to draw near to God with sincerity and humility, assuring us that as we do, God will draw near to us in return.

Drawing near to God involves more than just physical proximity; it's about the posture of our hearts. James highlights the importance of spiritual cleansing and purity. We're called to repentance, to turn away from sin and worldly distractions, and to purify our hearts, removing any double-mindedness or divided loyalty.

When we draw near to God, we open ourselves to His presence, His guidance, and His transformational power. It's in this closeness to Him that we find comfort, strength, and fulfillment beyond what the world can offer. God longs for a relationship with us, and as we respond to His invitation, He meets us with love, grace, and mercy.

DISCUSSION QUESTIONS

What are some practical ways we can draw near to God in our daily lives?

How does sin and spiritual impurity hinder our relationship with God, and what steps can we take to address them and more towards holiness?

Reflecting on James 4:8, what does it mean to you personally to have God draw near to you?

How can we maintain a consistent and authentic relationship with God amidst the busyness and distractions of life?

In what ways can we encourage one another to pursue intimacy with God within our Christian community?

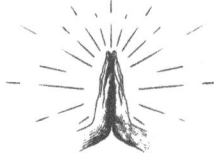

PRAYER

Heavenly Father, we are grateful for the invitation to draw near to you. Help us to approach you with sincere hearts, seeking intimacy and communion with you. Forgive us for our sins and cleanse us from all impurity. May we continually strive to purify our hearts and minds, aligning them with your will and purposes. Thank you for the promise that as we draw near to you, you will draw near to us. May our relationship with you deepen and flourish each day. In Jesus' name, we pray, Amen.

WEEK 2:
PRAYER AND COMMUNICATION

JAMES 5:16 (NIV)

"Therefore confess your sins to each other and pray for each other so that you may be healed. The prayer of a righteous person is powerful and effective."

DEVOTION

Prayer is a powerful tool for deepening our connection with God and fostering meaningful communication with Him. James 5:16 highlights the transformative nature of prayer, emphasizing its effectiveness in bringing healing and restoration to both individuals and communities.

The verse begins with an exhortation to confess sins and pray for one another. Confession opens the door to authenticity and vulnerability in our relationships, both with God and with fellow believers. When we confess our sins to God, we acknowledge our need for His forgiveness and restoration. Moreover, when we pray for one another, we demonstrate love and solidarity within the body of Christ, lifting each other up in prayer and interceding on behalf of our brothers and sisters.

James goes on to affirm the power and effectiveness of prayer, particularly the prayer of a righteous person. Righteousness is not merely a matter of outward behavior but also of a heart surrendered to God. The prayer of a righteous person is characterized by faith, fervency, and alignment with God's will. It is not the eloquence of words but the sincerity of heart that makes prayer powerful and effective.

Prayer is not a passive activity but an active engagement with the divine. It is a spiritual discipline that requires intentionality, perseverance, and faith. Through prayer, we invite God to work in our lives and in the lives of others, trusting in His wisdom and sovereignty.

The promise of healing in this verse encompasses not only physical healing but also emotional, relational, and spiritual healing. Prayer has the power to bring about transformation and restoration in every area of our lives. It is a means of experiencing God's grace, mercy, and healing touch.

As we embrace the practice of confession and prayer, may we experience the transformative power of God's presence in our lives and communities. Let us draw near to Him with confidence, knowing that our prayers are heard and that He delights in responding to the cries of His children.

DISCUSSION QUESTIONS

How does confession and prayer contribute to fostering authentic relationships within the body of Christ?

Can you share a personal testimony of how prayer has brought healing or restoration in your life or in the life of someone you know?

What does it mean to pray fervently and with faith? How can we cultivate these qualities in our prayer life?

In what ways can we support and encourage one another in our prayer lives within our families, small groups, or church communities?

How can we remain steadfast in prayer, even when we do not see immediate answers or outcomes?

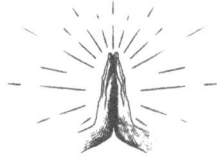

PRAYER

Heavenly Father, we thank you for the privilege of prayer. Help us to approach you with confidence, knowing that you are a loving and attentive God who hears our prayers. Grant us the wisdom to surrender our anxieties and concerns to you, trusting in your provision and sovereignty. May your peace, which surpasses all understanding, guard our hearts and minds in Christ Jesus. In Jesus' name, we pray, Amen.

WEEK 3:
STUDYING SCRIPTURE

2 TIMOTHY 3:16-17 (NIV)

"All Scripture is God-breathed and is useful for teaching, rebuking, correcting and training in righteousness, so that the servant of God may be thoroughly equipped for every good work."

DEVOTION

The Bible, as the inspired Word of God, holds immeasurable value and significance in the life of every believer. In 2 Timothy 3:16-17, Paul affirms the divine origin and practical application of Scripture. He emphasizes that all Scripture is God-breathed and serves a vital purpose in our spiritual growth and maturity.

Studying Scripture goes beyond mere intellectual pursuit; it's about encountering the living God and allowing His Word to transform our hearts and lives. Through the Bible, God teaches us His truth, convicts us of sin, corrects our misunderstandings, and trains us in righteousness. It equips us to live out our faith effectively, enabling us to fulfill God's purposes and engage in every good work He has prepared for us.

As we immerse ourselves in Scripture, we are drawn into a deeper understanding of God's character, His promises, and His will for our lives. It serves as a lamp to our feet and a light to our path, guiding us in the midst of life's uncertainties and challenges. Studying God's Word empowers us to walk in obedience, to resist temptation, and to grow in intimacy with our Heavenly Father.

DISCUSSION QUESTIONS

What are some practical strategies for cultivating a habit of studying Scripture regularly?

How has studying the Bible impacted your personal growth and relationship with God?

In what ways does Scripture challenge and convict us in our daily lives?

How can we ensure that our study of Scripture leads to transformation and application, rather than just acquiring knowledge?

How can we encourage and support one another in our journey of studying and applying God's Word within our Christian community?

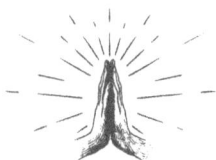

PRAYER

Heavenly Father, we thank you for the gift of your Word. Help us to approach Scripture with reverence and humility, recognizing its authority and power in our lives. Open our hearts and minds to receive your truth and wisdom as we study your Word. May it penetrate deep within us, transforming us from the inside out and equipping us for every good work you have prepared for us. Guide us by your Spirit as we seek to apply what we learn, living lives that honor and glorify you. In Jesus' name, we pray, Amen.

WEEK 4:
WORSHIP AND PRAISE

PSALM 95:1-2 (NIV)

"Come, let us sing for joy to the Lord; let us shout aloud to the Rock of our salvation. Let us come before him with thanksgiving and extol him with music and song."

DEVOTION

Psalm 95 beautifully captures the essence of worship and praise—a response of joy, gratitude, and adoration towards our God. It invites us to join together in lifting our voices and hearts in exultant praise to the Rock of our salvation.

Worship is not confined to a specific time or place but is a lifestyle characterized by a heart posture of reverence and awe towards God. It encompasses not only our songs and melodies but also our thoughts, actions, and attitudes. As we come before God with thanksgiving and praise, we acknowledge His sovereignty, faithfulness, and goodness in our lives.

In worship, we encounter the presence of God in a profound way. It's a divine exchange where we offer our praises to Him, and in return, He fills us with His peace, joy, and strength. Worship has the power to transform us from the inside out, aligning our hearts with God's purposes and drawing us into deeper intimacy with Him.

DISCUSSION QUESTIONS

How do you personally define worship, and what role does it play in your relationship with God?

Reflecting on Psalm 95:1-2, why is it important for believers to come together in corporate worship?

In what ways does worshiping God with gratitude and praise impact our perspective on life's challenges and blessings?

How can we cultivate a lifestyle of worship beyond Sunday gatherings, incorporating it into our daily routines?

What are some practical ways we can encourage one another to engage in heartfelt worship within our Christian community?

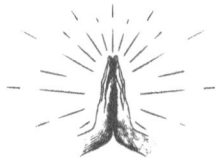

PRAYER

Heavenly Father, we are grateful for the privilege of worshiping you. Help us to approach you with hearts full of gratitude and praise, recognizing your greatness and faithfulness in our lives. May our worship be pleasing to you, drawing us into deeper intimacy with you and transforming us to reflect your love and character to the world. Guide us by your Spirit as we seek to exalt you in every area of our lives. In Jesus' name, we pray, Amen.

WEEK 5:

FELLOWSHIP WITH BELIEVERS

HEBREWS 10:24-25 (NIV)

"And let us consider how we may spur one another on toward love and good deeds, not giving up meeting together, as some are in the habit of doing, but encouraging one another—and all the more as you see the Day approaching."

DEVOTION

In Hebrews 10:24-25, we are reminded of the importance of fellowship within the body of Christ. As believers, we are called to actively engage with one another, encouraging and uplifting each other in our faith journey. This passage highlights three key aspects of fellowship: encouragement, accountability, and mutual support.

Firstly, fellowship provides us with encouragement. It's a place where we can find solace and strength amidst life's challenges, knowing that we are not alone in our struggles. Through genuine relationships with fellow believers, we receive words of affirmation, comfort, and hope, spurring us on towards love and good deeds.

Secondly, fellowship fosters accountability. As we gather together, we have the opportunity to hold each other accountable in our walk with God. We can lovingly challenge one another to live in alignment with God's Word, to pursue holiness, and to strive for excellence in all aspects of our lives.

Finally, fellowship offers mutual support. In times of celebration or sorrow, our Christian community stands by our side, offering prayers, practical assistance, and a listening ear. Together, we share in each other's joys and burdens, embodying the love and compassion of Christ.

As the day of Christ's return draws near, the need for fellowship becomes even more crucial. It's a time for us to rally together, to strengthen our bonds of unity, and to continue spurring one another on towards love and good deeds.

DISCUSSION QUESTIONS

What does fellowship mean to you, and how has it impacted your spiritual journey?

Reflecting on Hebrews 10:24-25, why is it important for believers to gather regularly and not forsake meeting together?

How can we effectively encourage one another in our Christian walk within our community?

In what ways does fellowship contribute to our growth in love and good deeds?

How can we overcome barriers to fellowship, such as busyness or social discomfort, within our church or small group settings?

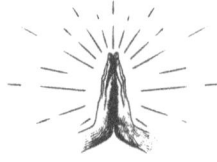

PRAYER

Gracious God, we thank you for the gift of fellowship within the body of Christ. Help us to cherish and nurture the relationships we have with fellow believers, recognizing the vital role they play in our spiritual growth and well-being. Guide us to be sources of encouragement, accountability, and support to one another, so that together, we may glorify you and advance your kingdom. In Jesus' name, we pray, Amen.

WEEK 6:

SURRENDER AND OBEDIENCE

ROMANS 12:1-2 (NIV)

"Therefore, I urge you, brothers and sisters, in view of God's mercy, to offer your bodies as a living sacrifice, holy and pleasing to God—this is your true and proper worship. Do not conform to the pattern of this world, but be transformed by the renewing of your mind. Then you will be able to test and approve what God's will is—his good, pleasing and perfect will."

DEVOTION

Romans 12:1-2 calls us to a life of surrender and obedience to God. It begins with an urgent plea, grounded in the understanding of God's mercy toward us. In response to His immense love and grace, we are called to present ourselves as living sacrifices—fully devoted and consecrated to God's purposes.

Surrendering to God involves yielding our will, desires, and ambitions to His sovereign authority. It requires a willingness to lay down our own plans and preferences, trusting in God's wisdom and guidance. Surrender is not a one-time event but a daily posture of humility and submission before our Heavenly Father.

Obedience is the natural outflow of surrender. As we yield ourselves to God, our lives are transformed. We are no longer conformed to the patterns of this world but are renewed in our minds by the truth of God's Word and the work of His Spirit within us. This transformation empowers us to discern and obey God's will, which is good, pleasing, and perfect.

True worship, according to this passage, is found in surrender and obedience. It's not merely about rituals or outward expressions but about the condition of our hearts and our willingness to align our lives with God's purposes.

DISCUSSION QUESTIONS

What does it mean to you to offer your life as a living sacrifice to God?

How does the concept of surrender challenge our natural inclination for control and self-reliance?

Reflecting on Romans 12:1-2, how can we actively resist conformity to the world's values and instead be transformed by God's truth?

In what areas of your life do you struggle the most with surrender and obedience to God?

How can we support and encourage one another in our journey of surrender and obedience within our Christian community?

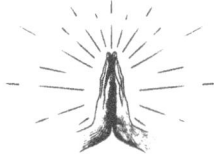

PRAYER

Heavenly Father, we thank you for your mercy and grace toward us. Help us to live lives of surrender and obedience, offering ourselves as living sacrifices, holy and pleasing to you. Renew our minds by your Spirit, that we may discern and follow your will in all things. Give us the strength and courage to resist conformity to the world and to walk in obedience to your Word. May our lives be a true reflection of worship, honoring and glorifying you in everything we do. In Jesus' name, we pray, Amen.

WEEK 7:
FORGIVENESS AND REPENTANCE

1 JOHN 1:9 (NIV)

"If we confess our sins, he is faithful and just and will forgive us our sins and purify us from all unrighteousness."

DEVOTION

1 John 1:9 beautifully encapsulates the essence of forgiveness and repentance. It serves as a comforting reminder of God's faithfulness and justice, and His willingness to forgive us when we humbly confess our sins. This verse underscores the transformative power of forgiveness and repentance in our lives.

Forgiveness is a central theme in the message of the Gospel. God's love for us is so immense that He sent His Son, Jesus Christ, to die for our sins, offering us the gift of forgiveness and reconciliation with Him. When we come to God with contrite hearts, acknowledging our sins and shortcomings, He graciously extends His forgiveness to us, wiping away our guilt and shame.

Repentance, likewise, is integral to our Christian walk. It involves a genuine turning away from sin and a sincere commitment to live in alignment with God's will. Repentance requires humility, as we acknowledge our need for God's mercy and grace. It's a transformative process that leads to spiritual renewal and growth, enabling us to experience the fullness of life that God desires for us.

As we embrace forgiveness and repentance, we are purified from all unrighteousness. Our relationship with God is restored, and we are empowered to live victoriously as children of God. Through the power of forgiveness and repentance, we find healing, restoration, and freedom from the bondage of sin.

DISCUSSION QUESTIONS

How do you personally understand the concept of forgiveness in light of 1 John 1:9?

Why is confession of sins an essential aspect of the Christian faith, and how does it contribute to spiritual growth?

Reflecting on 1 John 1:9, what are some barriers that may hinder people from confessing their sins and receiving God's forgiveness?

How can we cultivate a spirit of repentance in our daily lives, seeking to align ourselves with God's will?

In what ways can we extend the grace and forgiveness we have received from God to others in our relationships and interactions?

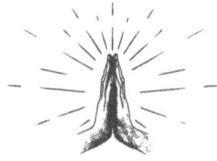

PRAYER

Heavenly Father, we thank you for your unfailing love and mercy towards us. Help us to embrace forgiveness and repentance as essential components of our faith journey. Give us the humility to confess our sins and the strength to turn away from them, trusting in your faithfulness to forgive us and purify us from all unrighteousness. May we walk in the freedom and joy of your forgiveness, extending grace and mercy to others as we have received from you. In Jesus' name, we pray, Amen.

WEEK 8:
SPIRITUAL WARFARE

EPHESIANS 6:10-18 (NIV)

"Finally, be strong in the Lord and in his mighty power. Put on the full armor of God, so that you can take your stand against the devil's schemes. For our struggle is not against flesh and blood, but against the rulers, against the authorities, against the powers of this dark world and against the spiritual forces of evil in the heavenly realms. Therefore put on the full armor of God, so that when the day of evil comes, you may be able to stand your ground, and after you have done everything, to stand. Stand firm then, with the belt of truth buckled around your waist, with the breastplate of righteousness in place, and with your feet fitted with the readiness that comes from the gospel of peace. In addition to all this, take up the shield of faith, with which you can extinguish all the flaming arrows of the evil one. Take the helmet of salvation and the sword of the Spirit, which is the word of God. And pray in the Spirit on all occasions with all kinds of prayers and requests. With this in mind, be alert and always keep on praying for all the Lord's people."

DEVOTION

The passage from Ephesians 6:10-18 paints a vivid picture of the spiritual battle we face as believers. It reminds us that our struggle is not against flesh and blood but against the spiritual forces of evil. In this warfare, we are called to be strong in the Lord and to put on the full armor of God.

The armor described in this passage symbolizes the spiritual resources and protections God provides for us to withstand the attacks of the enemy. Each piece of armor—truth, righteousness, the gospel of peace, faith, salvation, and the Word of God—equips us to stand firm against the schemes of the devil.

As we engage in spiritual warfare, prayer is our greatest weapon. Through prayer, we align ourselves with God's will, tap into His power, and invite His presence to go before us. It's through prayer that we access the strength, wisdom, and discernment needed to navigate the battles we face.

In the midst of spiritual warfare, we are reminded to be alert and vigilant. The enemy seeks to deceive, discourage, and distract us from God's truth and purposes. But as we remain rooted in God's Word, clothed in His armor, and fervent in prayer, we can stand firm and overcome every attack of the enemy.

DISCUSSION QUESTIONS

How do you perceive spiritual warfare, and in what ways have you personally experienced it in your life?

Reflecting on Ephesians 6:10-18, what significance do you find in each piece of the armor of God?

Why is prayer emphasized as a crucial aspect of spiritual warfare, and how has prayer strengthened your resilience in facing spiritual battles?

In what ways can the church community support believers in engaging in spiritual warfare and standing firm in faith?

How can we remain vigilant and discerning in recognizing the enemy's tactics and staying rooted in God's truth?

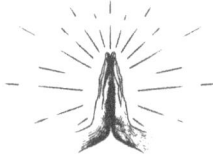

PRAYER

Heavenly Father, we thank you for the spiritual armor you provide for us to stand firm in the face of spiritual warfare. Equip us with strength and courage as we face the enemy's schemes. Help us to rely on your power, to stand firm in your truth, and to wield the sword of your Spirit, which is the Word of God. May our prayers be fervent, and may we remain vigilant and alert to the enemy's tactics. Grant us victory over every spiritual battle we encounter, for we know that in you, we are more than conquerors. In Jesus' name, we pray, Amen.

WEEK 9:

FRUIT OF THE SPIRIT

GALATIANS 5:22-23 (NIV)

"But the fruit of the Spirit is love, joy, peace, forbearance, kindness, goodness, faithfulness, gentleness and self-control. Against such things there is no law."

DEVOTION

In Galatians 5:22-23, Paul outlines the nine fruit of the Spirit, which are evidence of a life surrendered to God and filled with His presence. These characteristics reflect the nature of God Himself and serve as a testament to the transformative work of the Holy Spirit within believers.

- **Love:** Love is the foundational fruit of the Spirit, encompassing selfless devotion, compassion, and care for others.

- **Joy:** Joy is an abiding sense of gladness and contentment that transcends circumstances, rooted in our relationship with God.

- **Peace:** Peace is the assurance and tranquility that comes from trusting in God's sovereignty and resting in His promises.

- **Forbearance (Patience):** Forbearance is the ability to endure difficult situations and people with grace and patience, reflecting God's long-suffering nature.

- **Kindness:** Kindness involves showing genuine concern and consideration for others, extending mercy and grace as God has shown to us.

- **Goodness:** Goodness is the moral excellence and integrity that flows from a heart transformed by God's love.

- **Faithfulness:** Faithfulness is steadfastness and loyalty in our relationship with God and others, rooted in His unchanging nature.

- **Gentleness:** Gentleness is humility and meekness in our interactions with others, reflecting the gentleness and compassion of Christ.

- **Self-Control:** Self-control is the ability to govern our desires and impulses, surrendering to the guidance of the Holy Spirit.

As believers, we are called to cultivate this fruit in our lives through a continual dependence on God and a willingness to yield to His Spirit's leading. As we abide in Christ and allow His Spirit to work in us, we will bear fruit that glorifies God and blesses those around us.

DISCUSSION QUESTIONS

Which of the fruit of the Spirit do you find most challenging to cultivate in your life, and why?

How do the fruit of the Spirit differ from worldly virtues, and why is it important to distinguish between the two?

Reflecting on Galatians 5:22-23, how do you see the fruit of the Spirit manifested in the lives of believers around you?

In what practical ways can we intentionally cultivate the fruit of the Spirit in our daily lives?

How can the church community support and encourage one another in the journey of growing and bearing fruit in accordance with the Spirit?

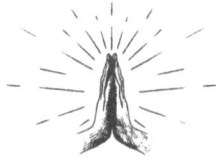

PRAYER

Heavenly Father, we thank you for the gift of your Spirit who enables us to bear fruit that reflects your character. Teach us to walk in step with your Spirit, yielding to His work in our lives. Help us to cultivate love, joy, peace, forbearance, kindness, goodness, faithfulness, gentleness, and self-control, that we may glorify you in all we do. May our lives be a testimony to your transforming power and grace. In Jesus' name, we pray, Amen.

WEEK 10:

SERVING OTHERS

1 PETER 4:10-11 (NIV)

"Each of you should use whatever gift you have received to serve others, as faithful stewards of God's grace in its various forms. If anyone speaks, they should do so as one who speaks the very words of God. If anyone serves, they should do so with the strength God provides, so that in all things God may be praised through Jesus Christ. To him be the glory and the power for ever and ever. Amen."

DEVOTION

In 1 Peter 4:10-11, Peter exhorts believers to utilize their spiritual gifts to serve others faithfully. He emphasizes that serving is not only a demonstration of God's grace in our lives but also an opportunity to glorify God through our actions.

As followers of Christ, we are called to be good stewards of the gifts and talents God has entrusted to us. Each of us has been uniquely equipped by God to contribute to the building up of His kingdom and the edification of His people. Whether it's through acts of service, words of encouragement, or sharing the gospel, we are to serve others wholeheartedly, recognizing that our ultimate aim is to bring glory to God.

Peter emphasizes the importance of serving with the strength God provides. Serving others can be demanding and challenging, but when we rely on God's strength and power, we are enabled to serve with joy and endurance. Our service becomes a testimony to God's faithfulness and a reflection of His love and compassion.

As we serve others with humility and grace, we embody the love of Christ and create spaces of hospitality and welcome. Through our words and deeds, we have the privilege of sharing God's grace with those around us, pointing them to the source of all goodness and mercy.

DISCUSSION QUESTIONS

How do you perceive the connection between serving others and being faithful stewards of God's grace, as described in 1 Peter 4:10-11?

What are some ways in which you have seen the strength of God manifest in your service to others?

Reflecting on your own spiritual gifts, how do you believe God has called you to serve others in your community or church?

In what practical ways can we cultivate a heart of hospitality and service in our daily lives?

How can we ensure that our motivation for serving others remains centered on bringing glory to God rather than seeking recognition or approval from others?

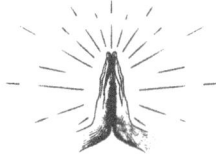

PRAYER

Gracious God, we thank you for the privilege of serving others as stewards of your grace. Help us to use our gifts and talents faithfully for the building up of your kingdom and the glory of your name. Grant us the strength and endurance to serve with joy and compassion, relying on your power and provision. May our words and deeds reflect your love and grace to all we encounter. To you be all the glory and praise forever and ever. Amen.

WEEK 11:

TRUST AND FAITH

PROVERBS 3:5-6 (NIV)

"Trust in the Lord with all your heart and lean not on your own understanding; in all your ways submit to him, and he will make your paths straight."

DEVOTION

Proverbs 3:5-6 offers a profound invitation to trust in the Lord wholeheartedly. It's a call to relinquish our own understanding and to submit to God's wisdom and guidance in every aspect of our lives. As we trust in Him, we experience His faithfulness and the assurance that He will direct our paths.

Trusting God with all our hearts means placing our confidence and reliance solely on Him, regardless of our circumstances or uncertainties. It involves surrendering our own plans and agendas, acknowledging that His ways are higher and His thoughts are beyond our comprehension. When we lean on our own understanding, we are limited by our finite perspective, but when we trust in God, we tap into His infinite wisdom and sovereignty.

In all our ways, we are called to submit to God—to yield our desires, decisions, and actions to His will. This submission requires humility and obedience, as we acknowledge God's authority over our lives and trust His plans, even when they diverge from our own.

As we journey in faith, trusting God's promises and guidance, He faithfully leads us along straight paths. Though the journey may be marked by twists and turns, challenges, and uncertainties, we can have confidence that God is with us, guiding us every step of the way.

DISCUSSION QUESTIONS

What does it mean to trust in the Lord with all your heart, and how does this differ from trusting in your own understanding?

Reflecting on Proverbs 3:5-6, why is it important to submit all aspects of our lives to God's will?

In what areas of your life do you find it most challenging to trust God completely? How can you cultivate a deeper trust in those areas?

How do you discern God's guidance and direction in your life amidst the noise and distractions of the world?

How can we support and encourage one another in our journey of trust and faith within our Christian community?

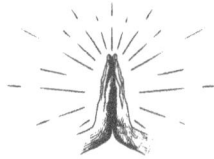

PRAYER

Heavenly Father, we thank you for your faithfulness and goodness towards us. Help us to trust in you with all our hearts, leaning not on our own understanding but acknowledging you in all our ways. Grant us the humility and obedience to submit to your will and guidance, trusting that you will make our paths straight. Strengthen our faith, Lord, and help us to rely on your wisdom and sovereignty in every aspect of our lives. In Jesus' name, we pray, Amen.

WEEK 12:

ENDURANCE AND PERSEVERANCE

HEBREWS 12:1-2 (NIV)

"Therefore, since we are surrounded by such a great cloud of witnesses, let us throw off everything that hinders and the sin that so easily entangles. And let us run with perseverance the race marked out for us, fixing our eyes on Jesus, the pioneer and perfecter of faith. For the joy set before him he endured the cross, scorning its shame, and sat down at the right hand of the throne of God."

DEVOTION

Hebrews 12:1-2 paints a vivid picture of the Christian life as a race—a journey of faith marked by endurance and perseverance. Just as athletes train rigorously and endure hardships to achieve victory, so too are believers called to run with perseverance the race marked out for them.

The author of Hebrews urges us to draw inspiration from the great cloud of witnesses who have gone before us—the faithful men and women of God whose lives testify to the power of endurance and perseverance in the face of trials and challenges. Their example encourages us to throw off everything that hinders us, including sin and distractions, and to press on towards the goal with determination.

Central to our endurance and perseverance is fixing our eyes on Jesus, the ultimate example of faithfulness and endurance. Jesus endured the cross, bearing the weight of our sins, out of love for us. His example inspires us to endure hardships and persevere in our faith journey, knowing that He is the pioneer and perfecter of our faith.

As we run the race of faith, we may encounter obstacles, trials, and setbacks along the way. But with our eyes fixed on Jesus, we can find strength, courage, and hope to press on. Our endurance and perseverance are not in vain, for they lead us to the ultimate prize—eternal life and communion with God.

DISCUSSION QUESTIONS

What are some hindrances or distractions that can impede our endurance and perseverance in the Christian life?

Reflecting on Hebrews 12:1-2, why is it important to draw inspiration from the examples of faithful witnesses who have gone before us?

How does fixing our eyes on Jesus help us to endure hardships and persevere in our faith journey?

Share about a time when you experienced God's strength and endurance in the midst of a trial or challenge.

In what practical ways can we encourage one another to persevere in the race of faith within our Christian community?

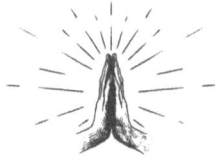

PRAYER

Heavenly Father, we thank you for the example of endurance and perseverance demonstrated by the faithful witnesses who have gone before us. Help us to throw off everything that hinders us and to run with perseverance the race marked out for us. May we fix our eyes on Jesus, the pioneer and perfecter of our faith, drawing strength and inspiration from His example. Grant us the grace to endure hardships and persevere in our faith journey, knowing that our ultimate prize is found in communion with you. In Jesus' name, we pray, Amen.

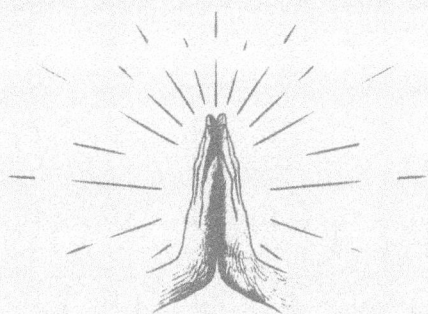

PHYSICAL HEALTH

TREATING YOUR BODY AS A TEMPLE

1 CORINTHIANS 6:19-20 (NIV)

"Do you not know that your bodies are temples of the Holy Spirit, who is in you, whom you have received from God? You are not your own; you were bought at a price. Therefore, honor God with your bodies."

DEVOTION

In 1 Corinthians 6:19-20, Paul reminds believers that their bodies are temples of the Holy Spirit. This profound truth carries significant implications for how we treat and care for our physical bodies. As temples of the Holy Spirit, our bodies are not our own; rather, they belong to God, having been purchased with the precious blood of Jesus Christ.

Treating our bodies as temples involves recognizing the sacredness and value that God has placed upon them. It means caring for our physical health and well-being, not out of vanity or selfishness, but out of reverence for the God who dwells within us. Just as we wouldn't defile a holy sanctuary, we are called to honor God with our bodies by living in a manner that reflects His holiness and righteousness.

This includes practicing self-discipline in areas such as diet, exercise, rest, and avoiding harmful substances. It also involves cultivating a positive body image, seeing ourselves as fearfully and wonderfully made in the image of God. Furthermore, it encompasses engaging in activities that promote spiritual, emotional, and mental well-being, recognizing that our bodies are interconnected with every aspect of our being.

By honoring God with our bodies, we not only demonstrate obedience and gratitude to Him but also bear witness to His transformative power in our lives. Our physical bodies become instruments through which we glorify God and fulfill His purposes in the world.

DISCUSSION QUESTIONS

How does the concept of treating your body as a temple challenge popular cultural attitudes towards physical health and self-care?

Reflecting on 1 Corinthians 6:19-20, why is it important for believers to recognize that their bodies belong to God?

In what practical ways can we honor God with our bodies in our daily lives?

Share about a time when you experienced the spiritual significance of caring for your physical health and well-being.

How can the church community support and encourage one another in cultivating a lifestyle that honors God with our bodies?

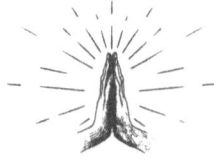

PRAYER

Heavenly Father, we thank you for the gift of our physical bodies, which you have entrusted to us as temples of your Holy Spirit. Help us to recognize the sacredness and value of our bodies and to honor you with them in all we do. Grant us the wisdom and discipline to care for our physical health and well-being, not for our own sake but for your glory. May our lives be a reflection of your holiness and love, as we seek to honor you with every aspect of our being. In Jesus' name, we pray, Amen.

WEEK 14:

PRACTICING MODERATION

PHILIPPIANS 4:5 (NIV)

"Let your gentleness be evident to all. The Lord is near."

DEVOTION

Philippians 4:5 encourages believers to let their gentleness or moderation be evident to all. This verse serves as a reminder of the importance of practicing moderation in all aspects of life. As followers of Christ, we are called to live balanced and temperate lives, avoiding extremes and excesses.

Practicing moderation involves finding a middle ground in various areas of life, including our behaviors, attitudes, and choices. It means exercising self-control and restraint, not allowing ourselves to be consumed by worldly desires or indulgences. Instead, we seek to maintain a balanced and harmonious approach to life, guided by the principles of God's Word.

Moderation is especially important in areas such as our use of time, finances, relationships, and even in our consumption of food. When we live in moderation, we demonstrate wisdom, discipline, and stewardship of the resources and blessings God has entrusted to us. We also reflect the character of Christ, who lived a life of humility, selflessness, and moderation.

By practicing moderation, we guard against the pitfalls of excess and imbalance, which can lead to stress, discontentment, and spiritual drift. Instead, we experience the freedom and peace that come from living in alignment with God's will and purposes for our lives.

DISCUSSION QUESTIONS

How do you understand the concept of moderation in the context of Philippians 4:5?

Reflecting on your own life, in what areas do you find it most challenging to practice moderation?

What are some potential consequences of living in excess or imbalance, and how does moderation help to mitigate these risks?

Share about a time when you experienced the benefits of practicing moderation in your life.

How can we encourage one another to live lives of moderation within our Christian community?

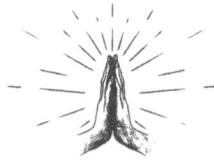

PRAYER

Heavenly Father, we thank you for the wisdom and guidance of your Word. Help us to live lives of moderation, finding balance and temperance in all things. Grant us the strength and discipline to exercise self-control and restraint, resisting the pull of excess and indulgence. May our lives be a reflection of your character, marked by gentleness, wisdom, and moderation. In Jesus' name, we pray, Amen.

WEEK 15:
REST AND SABBATH

MARK 2:27-28 (NIV)

"Then he said to them, 'The Sabbath was made for man, not man for the Sabbath. So the Son of Man is Lord even of the Sabbath.'"

DEVOTION

In Mark 2:27-28, Jesus teaches us about the significance of rest and the Sabbath. He reminds us that the Sabbath was not intended to be a burdensome obligation but a gift from God for our well-being and renewal. As the Lord of the Sabbath, Jesus invites us to embrace rest as an essential aspect of our lives.

Rest is not merely physical relaxation or cessation of activity but a holistic rejuvenation of our body, mind, and spirit. It involves withdrawing from our daily routines and responsibilities to seek refreshment and restoration in God's presence. The Sabbath, in particular, provides us with a designated time to pause, reflect, and reconnect with God and with our loved ones.

When we neglect rest, we risk burnout, exhaustion, and diminished spiritual vitality. Rest allows us to recharge and refocus, enabling us to live with greater intentionality and purpose. It reminds us of our dependence on God's provision and sovereignty, as we trust Him to sustain us even as we rest in Him.

As followers of Christ, we are called to honor the Sabbath and prioritize rest in our lives. This means setting aside time for intentional rest and rejuvenation, as well as cultivating a rhythm of rest in our daily lives. By embracing rest, we honor God's design for our well-being and demonstrate our trust in His care and provision.

DISCUSSION QUESTIONS

How do you currently prioritize rest and Sabbath in your life, and what challenges do you face in doing so?

Reflecting on Mark 2:27-28, why do you think Jesus emphasized the importance of rest and the Sabbath?

In what ways does rest contribute to our spiritual growth and well-being?

Share about a time when you experienced the benefits of intentional rest and Sabbath observance in your life.

How can we support and encourage one another in embracing rest and Sabbath within our Christian community?

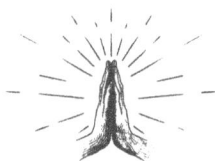

PRAYER

Heavenly Father, we thank you for the gift of rest and the Sabbath, which you have provided for our renewal and well-being. Help us to honor the Sabbath and prioritize rest in our lives, trusting in your provision and sovereignty. Grant us the wisdom to cultivate a rhythm of rest in our daily lives, that we may experience the fullness of life you intend for us. May our times of rest draw us closer to you and strengthen us for the journey ahead. In Jesus' name, we pray, Amen.

WEEK 16:

EXERCISE AND DISCIPLINE

1 TIMOTHY 4:8 (NIV)

"For physical training is of some value, but godliness has value for all things, holding promise for both the present life and the life to come."

DEVOTION

In 1 Timothy 4:8, Paul highlights the importance of both physical training and spiritual discipline. He acknowledges that physical exercise has value, but he emphasizes that godliness holds eternal significance, impacting not only our present lives but also our eternal destinies.

Physical exercise and discipline play a crucial role in maintaining our physical health and well-being. Engaging in regular exercise helps us to strengthen our bodies, improve our fitness, and enhance our overall quality of life. It allows us to steward the bodies that God has entrusted to us and to honor Him with our physical health.

However, while physical training is valuable, it is ultimately temporal in nature. In contrast, spiritual discipline and godliness have eternal implications. Cultivating godliness through prayer, study of God's Word, worship, and service leads to spiritual growth and transformation, shaping our character and preparing us for eternity.

As followers of Christ, we are called to prioritize both physical and spiritual discipline. This involves finding a balance between caring for our physical bodies and nurturing our spirits. Just as we set aside time for physical exercise, we must also carve out time for spiritual disciplines, investing in our relationship with God and growing in godliness.

By embracing discipline in both realms, we experience holistic growth and well-being, honoring God with our bodies and our spirits.

DISCUSSION QUESTIONS

How do you currently prioritize physical exercise and spiritual discipline in your life, and what challenges do you face in doing so?

Reflecting on 1 Timothy 4:8, why is it important to maintain a balance between physical training and spiritual discipline?

In what ways can physical exercise contribute to our spiritual growth and well-being?

Share about a time when you experienced the benefits of physical exercise or spiritual discipline in your life.

How can we support and encourage one another in embracing both physical and spiritual discipline within our Christian community?

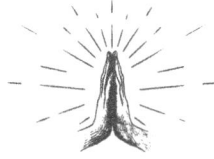

PRAYER

Heavenly Father, we thank you for the gift of physical health and spiritual growth. Help us to embrace discipline in both realms, prioritizing physical exercise and spiritual disciplines in our lives. Grant us the strength and motivation to care for our bodies and nurture our spirits, honoring you with all aspects of our being. May our pursuit of physical health and spiritual growth bring glory to your name and further your kingdom purposes. In Jesus' name, we pray, Amen.

WEEK 17:
PROPER NUTRITION

GENESIS 1:29 (NIV)

"Then God said, 'I give you every seed-bearing plant on the face of the whole earth and every tree that has fruit with seed in it. They will be yours for food.'"

DEVOTION

In Genesis 1:29, we see God's provision for nourishment as He grants humanity every seed-bearing plant and tree with fruit for food. This verse highlights the importance of proper nutrition, recognizing that God has provided us with a variety of foods to sustain and nourish our bodies.

As stewards of our bodies, it's essential for us to prioritize proper nutrition. God's provision of fruits, vegetables, grains, and other plant-based foods offers us a rich array of nutrients, vitamins, and minerals that promote health and well-being. By embracing a diet rich in whole, plant-based foods, we honor God's provision and care for our bodies.

Proper nutrition not only supports physical health but also influences our mental, emotional, and spiritual well-being. When we nourish our bodies with wholesome foods, we experience increased energy, vitality, and resilience. We are better equipped to serve God and others, fulfilling the purposes for which He has created us.

Moreover, choosing nutritious foods reflects our gratitude to God for His provision and stewardship of His creation. It's a tangible expression of our trust in His wisdom and care for us, as we partake in the bounty He has graciously provided.

DISCUSSION QUESTIONS

How does Genesis 1:29 inform our understanding of God's provision for proper nutrition?

Reflecting on your own eating habits, in what ways do you prioritize proper nutrition in your diet?

What are some practical benefits of embracing a diet rich in whole, plant-based foods?

Share about a time when you experienced the connection between proper nutrition and overall well-being in your life.

How can we support and encourage one another in making healthier dietary choices within our Christian community?

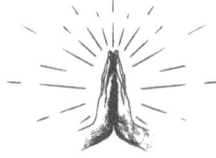

PRAYER

Heavenly Father, we thank you for your abundant provision of nourishing foods that sustain and strengthen our bodies. Help us to prioritize proper nutrition in our diets, honoring you with our choices and stewardship of our bodies. Grant us wisdom and discernment as we make decisions about what we eat, and may our dietary habits reflect our gratitude for your provision and care. May we be mindful of the connection between proper nutrition and our overall well-being, and may we glorify you in all that we do. In Jesus' name, we pray, Amen.

WEEK 18:

AVOIDING GLUTTONY

PROVERBS 23:20-21 (NIV)

"Do not join those who drink too much wine or gorge themselves on meat, for drunkards and gluttons become poor, and drowsiness clothes them in rags."

DEVOTION

Proverbs 23:20-21 provides wisdom regarding the dangers of gluttony and excessive consumption. Gluttony, characterized by overindulgence in food or drink, can lead to physical, spiritual, and financial consequences. As followers of Christ, we are called to exercise self-control and moderation in all aspects of our lives, including our eating habits.

Gluttony often stems from a lack of self-discipline and an improper relationship with food. Instead of viewing food as sustenance to fuel our bodies, we may turn to it for comfort, pleasure, or as a coping mechanism for stress or emotional issues. However, indulging in excessive eating or drinking sugary beverages can lead to negative consequences, including poor health, decreased productivity, and strained relationships.

As stewards of our bodies, it's essential to prioritize self-control and moderation in our eating habits. This involves being mindful of what and how much we consume, listening to our bodies' hunger and fullness cues, and making healthy choices that honor God and promote our well-being. By exercising self-control in our eating habits, we demonstrate obedience to God and respect for His gift of life and health.

Furthermore, resisting gluttony allows us to experience greater freedom and joy in our relationship with God. When we rely on His strength and guidance to overcome temptations, we grow in spiritual maturity and intimacy with Him. Our obedience in the area of self-control reflects our desire to honor God with every aspect of our lives, including our physical bodies.

DISCUSSION QUESTIONS

How does Proverbs 23:20-21 caution against the dangers of gluttony and excessive consumption?

Reflecting on your own eating habits, in what areas do you struggle with practicing self-control and moderation?

What are some practical strategies for resisting gluttony and cultivating a lifestyle of moderation in our eating habits?

Share about a time when you experienced the consequences of overindulgence or lack of self-control in your life.

How can we support and encourage one another in practicing self-control and moderation within our Christian community?

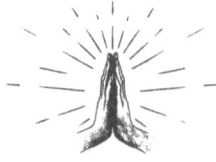

PRAYER

Heavenly Father, we thank you for the gift of food and nourishment that sustains our bodies. Help us to resist the temptation of gluttony and to exercise self-control and moderation in our eating habits. Grant us wisdom and strength to make healthy choices that honor you and promote our well-being. May our obedience in the area of self-control reflect our desire to honor you with every aspect of our lives. In Jesus' name, we pray, Amen.

FLEEING SEXUAL IMMORALITY

1 CORINTHIANS 6:18-19 (NIV)

"Flee from sexual immorality. All other sins a person commits are outside the body, but whoever sins sexually, sins against their own body. Do you not know that your bodies are temples of the Holy Spirit, who is in you, whom you have received from God? You are not your own;"

DEVOTION

In 1 Corinthians 6:18-19, Paul exhorts believers to flee from sexual immorality, emphasizing the sacredness and significance of our bodies as temples of the Holy Spirit. Sexual immorality not only defiles our bodies but also dishonors God, who has called us to purity and holiness.

As followers of Christ, we are called to uphold the sanctity of our bodies and our sexuality. God designed sex to be enjoyed within the bounds of marriage, as a sacred union between husband and wife. Any form of sexual activity outside of marriage—whether it be adultery, fornication, pornography, or lustful thoughts—violates God's design and undermines His purposes for human sexuality.

Sexual immorality not only harms us physically, emotionally, and spiritually but also damages our relationship with God and others. It distorts our understanding of love, intimacy, and commitment, leading to brokenness and heartache. By fleeing from sexual immorality, we honor God with our bodies and demonstrate our obedience to His commands.

Moreover, recognizing our bodies as temples of the Holy Spirit compels us to steward them with care and reverence. Just as we wouldn't defile a holy sanctuary, we must guard against anything that defiles our bodies, including sexual sin. We are called to present our bodies as living sacrifices, holy and pleasing to God, as an act of worship (Romans 12:1).

DISCUSSION QUESTIONS

What are some examples of sexual immorality in today's culture, and how do they conflict with biblical standards of purity?

How does the recognition of our bodies as temples of the Holy Spirit influence our approach to sexual purity?

What are some practical steps we can take to flee from sexual immorality and pursue purity in our lives?

Share about a time when you faced temptation or struggled with sexual immorality, and how God helped you overcome it.

How can we support and encourage one another in maintaining sexual purity within our Christian community?

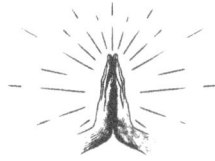

PRAYER

Heavenly Father, we thank you for the gift of sexuality and the sacredness of our bodies as temples of the Holy Spirit. Help us to flee from sexual immorality and to pursue purity and holiness in our thoughts, words, and actions. Give us strength and discernment to resist temptation and to honor you with our bodies. May our lives be a reflection of your holiness and love, as we seek to live in obedience to your commands. In Jesus' name, we pray, Amen.

WEEK 20:

SEEKING PHYSICAL HEALING

JAMES 5:14-15 (NIV)

"Is anyone among you sick? Let them call the elders of the church to pray over them and anoint them with oil in the name of the Lord. And the prayer offered in faith will make the sick person well; the Lord will raise them up. If they have sinned, they will be forgiven."

DEVOTION

James 5:14-15 offers guidance to believers who are in need of physical healing. It encourages them to seek the support and prayers of the church community, trusting in the power of God to bring about healing and restoration. This passage highlights the importance of faith-filled prayer and the role of the faith community in supporting those who are sick.

When facing illness or suffering, it can be tempting to rely solely on medical treatments or human interventions. However, James reminds us that our ultimate source of healing is God Himself. He is the Great Physician who has the power to heal both body and soul. By calling upon the elders of the church to pray over them and anoint them with oil, individuals demonstrate their trust in God's sovereignty and willingness to seek His intervention in their lives.

The promise of James 5:15 assures us that the prayer offered in faith will make the sick person well. While physical healing may not always occur in the manner or timing we expect, we can have confidence that God hears our prayers and works all things together for the good of those who love Him (Romans 8:28). Whether healing comes through miraculous intervention, medical treatment, or the comfort of His presence in the midst of suffering, we can trust in God's goodness and faithfulness.

Furthermore, James highlights the spiritual dimension of healing, emphasizing that if the sick person has sinned, they will be forgiven. Healing involves not only the restoration of physical health but also the reconciliation of our relationship with God. Through the healing process, God offers the gift of forgiveness and spiritual renewal, inviting us into deeper intimacy with Him.

DISCUSSION QUESTIONS

How does James 5:14-15 challenge our understanding of healing and the role of faith in the process?

Reflecting on your own experiences, how have you witnessed the power of faith-filled prayer in bringing about healing?

What are some obstacles or doubts that may hinder our faith when seeking healing?

Share about a time when you or someone you know experienced healing, either physically or spiritually, through prayer and faith.

How can the church community better support and pray for those who are in need of healing?

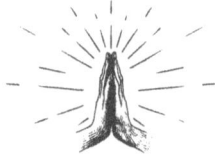

PRAYER

Heavenly Father, we thank you for your promise of healing and restoration. Give us faith to trust in your power and goodness, especially in times of illness or suffering. May we rely on the support and prayers of our faith community, knowing that you are the source of all healing. Grant us the grace to surrender our doubts and fears to you, and to trust in your perfect timing and purposes. In Jesus' name, we pray, Amen.

WEEK 21:

HYGIENE AND CLEANLINESS

LEVITICUS 11:44-45 (NIV)

"I am the Lord your God; consecrate yourselves and be holy, because I am holy. Do not make yourselves unclean by any creature that moves along the ground. I am the Lord, who brought you up out of Egypt to be your God; therefore be holy, because I am holy."

DEVOTION

In Leviticus 11:44-45, God commands His people to be holy, for He is holy. This call to holiness extends to all aspects of life, including personal hygiene and cleanliness. God's desire for His people to be holy encompasses not only spiritual purity but also physical cleanliness, reflecting the sacredness of their relationship with Him.

Maintaining proper hygiene and cleanliness is not only a matter of physical health but also a reflection of our reverence for God and His creation. As stewards of our bodies, which are temples of the Holy Spirit (1 Corinthians 6:19), we are called to care for them with diligence and respect. Practicing good hygiene helps to prevent the spread of disease, promote overall well-being, and honor the sanctity of our bodies as gifts from God.

Furthermore, cleanliness carries symbolic significance in the Bible, representing purity, righteousness, and consecration. Just as the Israelites were instructed to purify themselves before coming into the presence of God, so too are we called to cleanse ourselves from impurity and sin, both outwardly and inwardly. Our commitment to cleanliness reflects our desire to live holy lives, set apart for God's purposes.

DISCUSSION QUESTIONS

How does Leviticus 11:44-45 emphasize the connection between holiness and cleanliness?

Reflecting on your own habits, how do you prioritize personal hygiene and cleanliness in your daily life?

In what ways can maintaining cleanliness be an act of worship and obedience to God?

Share about a time when you experienced the spiritual significance of cleanliness in your life.

How can we encourage one another to cultivate habits of cleanliness and holiness within our Christian community?

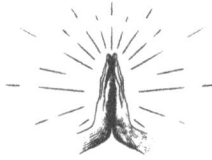

PRAYER

Heavenly Father, we thank you for the gift of cleanliness and hygiene, which promote health and well-being. Help us to honor you with our bodies by practicing good hygiene and cleanliness in our daily lives. May our commitment to cleanliness be a reflection of our desire to live holy and consecrated lives, set apart for your purposes. Grant us the grace to cultivate habits of cleanliness and holiness, that we may glorify you in all that we do. In Jesus' name, we pray, Amen.

WEEK 22:

CARING FOR THE VULNERABLE

JAMES 1:27 (NIV)

"Religion that God our Father accepts as pure and faultless is this: to look after orphans and widows in their distress and to keep oneself from being polluted by the world."

DEVOTION

James 1:27 encapsulates the essence of true religion in God's eyes: caring for the vulnerable. In this verse, we are called to extend compassion and support to those who are marginalized, including orphans and widows. This command reflects God's heart for the vulnerable and emphasizes the importance of demonstrating His love through practical acts of kindness and care.

Caring for the vulnerable is not merely an optional aspect of our faith but an integral part of living out the gospel. Jesus Himself demonstrated compassion and concern for the marginalized, reaching out to the outcasts, the sick, and the oppressed. As His followers, we are called to imitate His example, showing love and mercy to those in need.

The vulnerable among us include not only orphans and widows but also the elderly, the homeless, the impoverished, and the marginalized. They are individuals who may be facing various challenges and struggles, ranging from physical needs to emotional and spiritual distress. By extending a helping hand and offering support, we demonstrate Christ's love in tangible ways and bring hope to those who are in difficult circumstances.

Moreover, caring for the vulnerable is a reflection of our commitment to live lives that are "unpolluted by the world." It involves rejecting the selfish values of society and embracing God's kingdom values of love, justice, and compassion. As we seek to keep ourselves pure and blameless before God, we actively engage in acts of service and compassion towards the vulnerable, reflecting the transformative power of the gospel in our lives.

DISCUSSION QUESTIONS

How does James 1:27 challenge our understanding of true religion and the practice of our faith?

Reflecting on your own life, in what ways do you currently engage in caring for the vulnerable?

Who are some vulnerable groups in your community, and how can you extend care and support to them?

Share about a time when you witnessed the impact of caring for the vulnerable, either personally or through others' actions.

How can we as a church community actively engage in caring for the vulnerable and living out James 1:27?

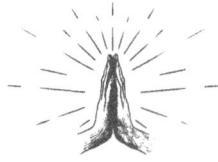

PRAYER

Heavenly Father, we thank you for your heart of compassion and love for the vulnerable. Help us to embody the spirit of James 1:27, reaching out to those who are marginalized and in need. Give us wisdom and discernment to identify opportunities to extend care and support to the vulnerable in our communities. May our actions reflect your love and bring glory to your name. In Jesus' name, we pray, Amen.

WEEK 23:

AVOIDING SUBSTANCE ABUSE

PROVERBS 20:1 (NIV)

"Wine is a mocker and beer a brawler; whoever is led astray by them is not wise."

DEVOTION

Proverbs 20:1 offers a poignant warning against the dangers of substance abuse, highlighting the deceptive allure of alcohol and its potential to lead individuals astray. While alcohol itself is not inherently evil, its misuse and abuse can have devastating consequences on both individuals and society as a whole.

The imagery used in this verse paints a vivid picture of the negative effects of alcohol: wine is depicted as a mocker, and beer as a brawler. These substances have the potential to distort judgment, impair reasoning, and incite conflict. Those who are led astray by them are not acting in wisdom or exercising self-control.

As followers of Christ, we are called to walk in wisdom and self-control, resisting the temptations of substance abuse. This involves making intentional choices to safeguard our physical, mental, and spiritual well-being, and to avoid anything that may lead us down a destructive path. That may include abstaining from alcohol all together so that we don't lead our brothers and sisters astray, as well.

Substance abuse not only harms individuals but also undermines relationships, compromises health, and contributes to societal problems such as crime and violence. By choosing sobriety, we demonstrate our commitment to honoring God with our bodies and minds, and to living lives that reflect His wisdom and righteousness.

DISCUSSION QUESTIONS

How does Proverbs 20:1 caution against the dangers of substance abuse and its negative effects?

Reflecting on your own experiences or observations, what are some consequences of substance abuse in individuals' lives and in society?

In what ways can we cultivate wisdom and self-control to resist the temptation of substance abuse?

Share about a time when you or someone you know faced the temptation of substance abuse and how you navigated it.

How can we support and encourage one another in making healthy choices and avoiding substance abuse within our Christian community?

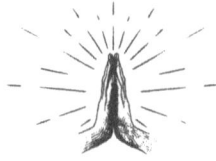

PRAYER

Heavenly Father, we thank you for the gift of wisdom and self-control. Help us to heed the warning of Proverbs 20:1 and to avoid the dangers of substance abuse. Grant us strength and discernment to make healthy choices that honor you and promote our well-being. May we be a source of support and encouragement to one another in living lives of sobriety and righteousness. In Jesus' name, we pray, Amen.

WEEK 24:

SEEKING BALANCE

ECCLESIASTES 3:1-8 (NIV)

"There is a time for everything, and a season for every activity under the heavens: a time to be born and a time to die, a time to plant and a time to uproot, a time to kill and a time to heal, a time to tear down and a time to build, a time to weep and a time to laugh, a time to mourn and a time to dance, a time to scatter stones and a time to gather them, a time to embrace and a time to refrain from embracing, a time to search and a time to give up, a time to keep and a time to throw away, a time to tear and a time to mend, a time to be silent and a time to speak, a time to love and a time to hate, a time for war and a time for peace."

DEVOTION

Ecclesiastes 3:1-8 reminds us of the natural ebb and flow of life's seasons, each with its own unique rhythms and purposes. In this passage, we are presented with a series of contrasting activities and emotions, illustrating the diverse experiences we encounter throughout our lives. From birth to death, planting to uprooting, weeping to laughing, and everything in between, there is a time and a season for each.

Finding balance in life involves embracing these diverse seasons and learning to navigate the transitions with grace and wisdom. It means recognizing that each season has its own purpose and significance, whether it be a time of growth and abundance or a time of pruning and loss. By embracing the full spectrum of life's experiences, we gain a deeper appreciation for the richness and complexity of God's design.

Moreover, seeking balance requires discernment and intentionality in how we allocate our time, energy, and resources. Just as there is a time for work and a time for rest, there is also a time for service and a time for solitude, a time for productivity and a time for leisure. By prioritizing what matters most and aligning our actions with our values and priorities, we can live with greater purpose and fulfillment.

DISCUSSION QUESTIONS

How does Ecclesiastes 3:1-8 challenge our understanding of balance and the rhythms of life?

Reflecting on the various activities and emotions described in this passage, which ones resonate with you most at this season of your life?

In what areas of your life do you struggle to find balance, and what steps can you take to address this imbalance?

Share about a time when you experienced the importance of embracing a particular season or transition in your life.

How can we support and encourage one another in seeking balance and navigating life's seasons within our Christian community?

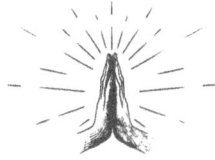

PRAYER

Heavenly Father, we thank you for the wisdom of Ecclesiastes 3:1-8, which reminds us of the diverse seasons and rhythms of life. Help us to embrace each season with grace and wisdom, trusting in your sovereign plan and purpose. Grant us discernment and intentionality as we seek balance in our lives, aligning our actions with your will and priorities. May we find fulfillment and joy in every season, knowing that you are with us every step of the way. In Jesus' name, we pray, Amen.

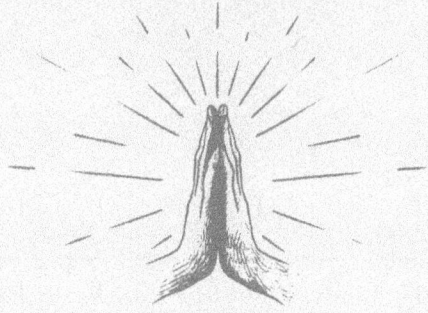

MENTAL HEALTH

WEEK 25:

TRUSTING IN GOD'S SOVEREIGNTY

PSALM 103:19 (NIV)

> *"The Lord has established his throne in heaven,*
> *and his kingdom rules over all."*

DEVOTION

As we journey through life, we often encounter situations that challenge our faith and understanding. In times of uncertainty, it's essential to anchor ourselves in the truth of God's sovereignty. Psalm 103:19 reminds us of the unwavering rule of our heavenly Father. It declares that the Lord has established His throne in heaven, and His kingdom rules over all. This verse invites us to reflect on the profound and comforting reality of God's sovereignty.

God's sovereignty means that He is in control of all things, both in heaven and on earth. Nothing happens outside of His knowledge, authority, or plan. Even when circumstances seem chaotic or beyond our comprehension, we can find peace in knowing that God reigns supreme over every situation. His sovereignty extends over the entire universe, from the grandest celestial bodies to the smallest details of our lives.

When we meditate on God's sovereignty, it shifts our perspective from fear and doubt to trust and confidence. We can trust in His wisdom, goodness, and faithfulness, knowing that He works all things together for our good and His glory (Romans 8:28). Instead of relying on our limited understanding, we can surrender to His perfect will and rest in His loving care.

In times of trial or adversity, remembering God's sovereignty provides us with strength and hope. It reminds us that our circumstances are not determined by chance or fate but by the purposeful hand of our sovereign God. Even when we face challenges that seem insurmountable, we can take comfort in the assurance that God is in control and His plans will ultimately prevail.

As we contemplate the truth of God's sovereignty, let us draw near to Him in prayer and worship. Let us surrender our fears, anxieties, and uncertainties at His feet, trusting in His unfailing love and power. May we find solace in His presence and peace in His sovereignty, knowing that He holds us securely in His hands.

DISCUSSION QUESTIONS

How does understanding God's sovereignty impact your perspective on difficult circumstances in your life?

Can you think of a time when you struggled to trust in God's sovereignty? How did you overcome that struggle?

In what ways can meditating on God's sovereignty deepen your relationship with Him?

How does God's sovereignty influence your prayers and petitions to Him?

What practical steps can you take to remind yourself of God's sovereignty daily and live with a greater sense of trust and confidence in Him?

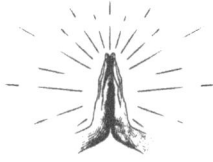

PRAYER

Heavenly Father, we thank you for your sovereignty and wisdom that surpasses all understanding. Help us to trust in you with all our hearts, leaning not on our own understanding but acknowledging your authority and power. Grant us the humility to submit to you in all our ways, surrendering our desires and plans to your will. May we find peace and assurance in knowing that you are in control, guiding us along the path of righteousness and blessing. In Jesus' name, we pray, Amen.

WEEK 26:
OVERCOMING ANXIETY

PHILIPPIANS 4:6-7 (NIV)

"Do not be anxious about anything, but in every situation, by prayer and petition, with thanksgiving, present your requests to God. And the peace of God, which transcends all understanding, will guard your hearts and your minds in Christ Jesus."

DEVOTION

Philippians 4:6-7 offers a powerful antidote to anxiety, providing a pathway to experience God's peace amidst life's uncertainties and challenges. In a world filled with stress and worry, this passage invites us to entrust our concerns to God through prayer and thanksgiving, confident in His ability to provide comfort, strength, and guidance.

Anxiety often stems from a sense of powerlessness and fear of the unknown. It can manifest in various forms, such as worry about the future, stress over circumstances beyond our control, or apprehension about potential outcomes. However, as believers, we are called to cast our anxieties upon the Lord, knowing that He cares for us and is able to carry our burdens.

The key to overcoming anxiety lies in surrendering our concerns to God through prayer and petition. Rather than dwelling on our worries or trying to solve problems in our own strength, we are invited to bring them to God in prayer, laying them at His feet and trusting in His provision and faithfulness. As we present our requests with thanksgiving, we shift our focus from our problems to the goodness and sovereignty of God, cultivating a heart of gratitude and trust.

Furthermore, the promise of Philippians 4:7 assures us that God's peace, which surpasses all understanding, will guard our hearts and minds in Christ Jesus. This peace is not dependent on our circumstances but is rooted in our relationship with God. It is a deep-seated assurance of His presence, His love, and His sovereign control over every aspect of our lives.

DISCUSSION QUESTIONS

How does Philippians 4:6-7 challenge our tendency to be anxious about the uncertainties of life?

Reflecting on your own experiences, what are some common triggers of anxiety in your life?

In what ways can prayer and thanksgiving help to alleviate anxiety and cultivate a sense of peace?

Share about a time when you experienced God's peace in the midst of a challenging situation or season of anxiety.

How can we support and encourage one another in overcoming anxiety and experiencing God's peace within our Christian community?

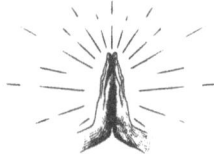

PRAYER

Heavenly Father, we thank you for the promise of your peace that surpasses all understanding. Help us to cast our anxieties upon you through prayer and thanksgiving, trusting in your provision and faithfulness. Grant us the strength to surrender our worries to you, knowing that you care for us deeply. May your peace guard our hearts and minds in Christ Jesus, enabling us to navigate life's uncertainties with confidence and trust in your unfailing love. In Jesus' name, we pray, Amen.

WEEK 27:

FINDING STRENGTH IN WEAKNESS

2 CORINTHIANS 12:9-10 (NIV)

"But he said to me, 'My grace is sufficient for you, for my power is made perfect in weakness.' Therefore, I will boast all the more gladly about my weaknesses, so that Christ's power may rest on me. That is why, for Christ's sake, I delight in weaknesses, in insults, in hardships, in persecutions, in difficulties. For when I am weak, then I am strong."

DEVOTION

2 Corinthians 12:9-10 offers profound insight into the paradoxical nature of strength and weakness in the Christian life. In this passage, the apostle Paul shares about his own experience of weakness and how God's grace and power were revealed through it. Rather than seeing weakness as a liability, Paul embraced it as an opportunity for God's strength to be displayed in his life.

As humans, we often strive to project an image of strength and self-sufficiency, fearing that vulnerability or weakness will be perceived as a sign of inadequacy. However, Paul's words remind us that our weaknesses do not disqualify us from experiencing God's power; rather, they provide a platform for His strength to be magnified.

God's grace is sufficient for us in our weakness. His power is made perfect in our moments of inadequacy, when we recognize our need for Him and rely fully on His strength. When we boast in our weaknesses, we acknowledge our dependency on Christ and invite His power to work in and through us.

Moreover, finding strength in weakness is not merely about enduring hardships or overcoming challenges through sheer willpower. It's about embracing our limitations and weaknesses, knowing that they draw us closer to God and deepen our reliance on His grace. In our moments of weakness, we discover the sufficiency of God's grace to sustain us and the transformative power of His Spirit to enable us to persevere.

DISCUSSION QUESTIONS

How does 2 Corinthians 12:9-10 challenge our cultural understanding of strength and weakness?

Reflecting on your own life, what are some weaknesses or limitations that you struggle with?

How can embracing weakness lead to a deeper experience of God's grace and power in your life?

Share about a time when you experienced God's strength in the midst of your weakness.

How can we encourage one another to embrace vulnerability and rely on God's strength within our Christian community?

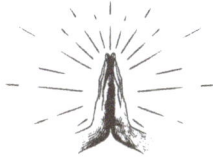

PRAYER

Heavenly Father, we thank you for the reminder that your grace is sufficient for us in our weakness. Help us to embrace our limitations and vulnerabilities, knowing that your power is made perfect in our moments of inadequacy. May we boast in our weaknesses, that Christ's power may rest on us and be magnified in our lives. Give us the strength to rely fully on your grace and to trust in your provision in every circumstance. In Jesus' name, we pray, Amen.

RENEWING THE MIND

ROMANS 12:2 (NIV)

"Do not conform to the pattern of this world, but be transformed by the renewing of your mind. Then you will be able to test and approve what God's will is—his good, pleasing and perfect will."

DEVOTION

Romans 12:2 emphasizes the importance of renewing our minds as a crucial aspect of our spiritual transformation. In a world filled with competing ideologies and values, it's easy to conform to the patterns and standards of society. However, as followers of Christ, we are called to a higher standard—to be transformed by the renewing of our minds.

Renewing our minds involves a deliberate and ongoing process of aligning our thoughts, attitudes, and beliefs with the truth of God's Word. It requires us to actively reject the influences of the world and instead immerse ourselves in the principles and teachings of Scripture. As we saturate our minds with God's truth, His Spirit works within us, reshaping our perspectives and guiding us into alignment with His will.

The transformation of our minds is not merely a cognitive exercise but a spiritual renewal that impacts every aspect of our lives. It changes the way we perceive ourselves, others, and the world around us. It enables us to discern God's will more clearly and to live in obedience to His purposes.

Moreover, renewing our minds empowers us to overcome the lies and deceptions of the enemy. It equips us to recognize and resist the temptations of sin, replacing old patterns of thinking with godly wisdom and discernment. As our minds are transformed, we become more effective witnesses for Christ, shining His light in a dark and broken world.

DISCUSSION QUESTIONS

How does Romans 12:2 challenge our tendency to conform to the patterns of this world?

Reflecting on your own life, what are some areas where your thinking needs to be renewed according to God's Word?

What are some practical ways we can engage in the process of renewing our minds on a daily basis?

Share about a time when renewing your mind through Scripture impacted your attitudes or behaviors.

How can we encourage one another to prioritize the renewal of our minds within our Christian community?

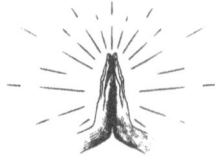

PRAYER

Heavenly Father, we thank you for the transformative power of your Word to renew our minds and hearts. Help us to resist the influence of the world and to immerse ourselves in the truth of Scripture. May your Spirit work within us to reshape our thinking and align it with your will. Grant us the wisdom and discernment to test and approve what is pleasing to you, and to live as faithful witnesses of your grace and truth. In Jesus' name, we pray, Amen.

WEEK 29:
SEEKING WISDOM

PROVERBS 4:7 (NIV)

"The beginning of wisdom is this: Get wisdom. Though it cost all you have, get understanding."

DEVOTION

Proverbs 4:7 succinctly encapsulates the essence of wisdom—the foundational importance of seeking understanding and insight. In a world filled with competing voices and conflicting ideologies, the pursuit of wisdom is essential for navigating life's complexities and making decisions that honor God.

Wisdom is more than mere knowledge or intelligence; it is the ability to discern truth, make sound judgments, and live in alignment with God's will. It involves seeking understanding, discerning right from wrong, and applying knowledge in practical ways that glorify God and benefit others.

The pursuit of wisdom requires intentionality and effort. It involves humility to recognize our need for guidance and instruction, and a willingness to seek wisdom diligently, even if it requires sacrifice. As the proverb states, "Though it cost all you have, get understanding." The value of wisdom far surpasses any material possession or earthly pursuit.

Moreover, wisdom is a lifelong journey—an ongoing process of growth and maturation. It is cultivated through a combination of studying God's Word, seeking counsel from wise mentors, and learning from life's experiences. As we walk in the fear of the Lord and apply His teachings to our lives, we grow in wisdom and understanding.

DISCUSSION QUESTIONS

What does Proverbs 4:7 teach us about the importance of seeking wisdom in our lives?

Reflecting on your own journey, how has the pursuit of wisdom impacted your decision-making and outlook on life?

In what areas of your life do you currently need wisdom and understanding?

Share about a time when seeking wisdom led to a significant decision or breakthrough in your life.

How can we cultivate a culture of wisdom-seeking within our Christian community?

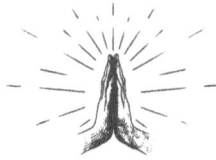

PRAYER

Heavenly Father, we thank you for the gift of wisdom and understanding. Help us to seek wisdom diligently, recognizing its surpassing value and importance in our lives. Grant us humility to acknowledge our need for guidance and instruction, and a willingness to pursue wisdom at all costs. May we walk in the fear of the Lord and apply His teachings to our lives, growing in wisdom and understanding each day. In Jesus' name, we pray, Amen.

WEEK 30:

ENCOURAGING ONE ANOTHER

1 THESSALONIANS 5:11 (NIV)

"Therefore encourage one another and build each other up, just as in fact you are doing."

DEVOTION

In 1 Thessalonians 5:11, Paul exhorts believers to encourage one another and build each other up. Encouragement is a powerful tool in the life of a Christian community—it strengthens bonds, uplifts spirits, and fosters a culture of love and support.

Encouragement involves more than just offering kind words; it's about affirming one another's value, potential, and contributions to the body of Christ. It's about standing alongside each other in both joys and sorrows, offering comfort, support, and hope.

As followers of Christ, we are called to be agents of encouragement in a world filled with discouragement and despair. Whether through a thoughtful word, a sincere compliment, or a simple act of kindness, we have the opportunity to make a positive difference in the lives of others.

Moreover, encouragement is reciprocal—often, as we encourage others, we ourselves are also uplifted. When we take the time to build each other up, we create a ripple effect of positivity and joy that extends far beyond ourselves.

DISCUSSION QUESTIONS

How does 1 Thessalonians 5:11 challenge us to prioritize encouragement in our interactions with others?

Reflecting on your own experiences, how has encouragement impacted your spiritual journey and relationships?

In what ways can we intentionally cultivate a culture of encouragement within our Christian community?

Share about a time when someone's encouragement made a significant difference in your life.

How can we encourage one another to persevere in faith and service, especially during challenging times?

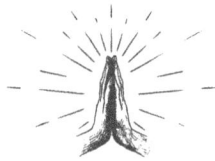

PRAYER

Heavenly Father, we thank you for the gift of encouragement and the power it holds to uplift and strengthen us. Help us to be agents of encouragement in our interactions with others, building each other up and fostering a culture of love and support within our Christian community. May our words and actions reflect your love and grace, bringing hope and joy to those around us. In Jesus' name, we pray, Amen.

WEEK 31:

CASTING OUR CARES ON GOD

1 PETER 5:7 (NIV)

"Cast all your anxiety on him because he cares for you."

DEVOTION

In 1 Peter 5:7, we are reminded of God's invitation to cast all our cares and anxieties upon Him. This verse acknowledges the reality of life's burdens and challenges but assures us of God's care and provision in the midst of them.

Casting our cares on God involves a deliberate act of surrender—releasing our worries, fears, and burdens into His capable hands. It requires trust in God's character and faithfulness, knowing that He is not only willing but also able to bear our burdens and provide for our needs.

Furthermore, the assurance that God cares for us is a comforting truth that brings hope and peace in times of trial. It reminds us that we are not alone in our struggles; God is intimately acquainted with our needs and is actively involved in every aspect of our lives.

As we cast our cares on God, we are freed from the heavy burden of anxiety and worry. We can rest in the assurance that God is in control and that His plans for us are good. This does not mean that we will be exempt from difficulties, but it does mean that we can face them with confidence, knowing that God is with us every step of the way.

DISCUSSION QUESTIONS

How does 1 Peter 5:7 encourage us to approach our cares and anxieties?

Reflecting on your own life, what are some cares or worries that you need to cast upon God?

In what ways can we practically cast our cares on God in our daily lives?

Share about a time when you experienced the peace and provision of God after casting your cares upon Him.

How can we encourage one another to trust in God's care and provision, especially during challenging times?

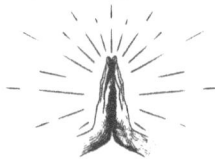

PRAYER

Heavenly Father, we thank you for the assurance that we can cast all our cares upon you because you care for us. Help us to surrender our anxieties and worries to you, trusting in your care and provision. Grant us the faith to believe that you are working all things together for our good, even in the midst of trials and uncertainties. May we find peace and rest in your loving embrace. In Jesus' name, we pray, Amen.

WEEK 32:
PRACTICING GRATITUDE

1 THESSALONIANS 5:18 (NIV)

"Give thanks in all circumstances; for this is God's will for you in Christ Jesus."

DEVOTION

In 1 Thessalonians 5:18, Paul instructs believers to give thanks in all circumstances. This call to gratitude is not contingent upon our circumstances but is a reflection of our trust in God's sovereignty and goodness. Practicing gratitude is a transformative spiritual discipline that shifts our focus from what we lack to what we have been given.

Gratitude is not merely a fleeting emotion but a deliberate choice—a posture of the heart that acknowledges God's blessings and provisions in our lives. It involves cultivating a spirit of thankfulness, even in the midst of trials and challenges, recognizing that God is at work in all things for our good.

Moreover, gratitude is an expression of faith and trust in God's faithfulness and provision. When we give thanks in all circumstances, we affirm our belief that God is in control and that His plans for us are good. Gratitude fosters humility, reminding us of our dependence on God and the generosity of His love and grace.

As we cultivate thankfulness in our lives, we experience a shift in perspective—a renewed sense of joy, contentment, and peace. Gratitude opens our eyes to the countless blessings that surround us each day, from the gift of salvation to the beauty of creation to the love of family and friends.

DISCUSSION QUESTIONS

How does 1 Thessalonians 5:18 challenge our understanding of gratitude and thanksgiving?

Reflecting on your own life, what are some blessings or reasons for gratitude that you often overlook?

In what ways can we practice gratitude in our daily lives, even in the midst of difficulties?

Share about a time when practicing gratitude transformed your perspective or brought joy in the midst of adversity.

How can we encourage one another to cultivate a spirit of gratitude within our Christian community?

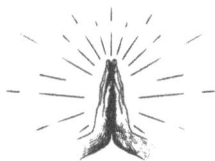

PRAYER

Heavenly Father, we thank you for the countless blessings you have bestowed upon us. Help us to cultivate a spirit of gratitude in our lives, giving thanks in all circumstances. Open our eyes to the abundance of your provision and the beauty of your creation. May our hearts overflow with thanksgiving, as we trust in your goodness and faithfulness. In Jesus' name, we pray, Amen.

WEEK 33:

FINDING REST IN GOD

MATTHEW 11:28-30 (NIV)

"Come to me, all you who are weary and burdened, and I will give you rest. Take my yoke upon you and learn from me, for I am gentle and humble in heart, and you will find rest for your souls. For my yoke is easy and my burden is light."

DEVOTION

In Matthew 11:28-30, Jesus extends a heartfelt invitation to all who are weary and burdened, promising them rest. This invitation is not merely physical rest but a deep, soul-satisfying rest that can only be found in God's presence.

The world we live in is filled with busyness, stress, and turmoil, often leaving us feeling exhausted and overwhelmed. We may find ourselves weighed down by the demands of work, family, relationships, or even our own expectations. In the midst of this chaos, Jesus offers us a place of refuge—a sanctuary of rest where we can find solace and renewal.

Finding rest in God involves surrendering our burdens and worries to Him, trusting in His provision and care. It means releasing our need for control and allowing God to take the reins of our lives. As we come to Him in humility and dependence, we discover the restorative power of His presence.

Moreover, Jesus invites us to take His yoke upon us and learn from Him. His yoke is not burdensome or oppressive but gentle and easy to bear. As we walk alongside Him, we find guidance, comfort, and strength for the journey. We learn from His example of humility and servanthood, and we experience firsthand the peace that comes from abiding in Him.

DISCUSSION QUESTIONS

How does Matthew 11:28-30 challenge our understanding of rest and burden-bearing?

Reflecting on your own life, what are some burdens or worries that you need to surrender to God?

In what ways can we practically come to Jesus and find rest for our souls in the midst of busy and stressful lives?

Share about a time when you experienced God's restorative presence in a moment of weariness or struggle.

How can we encourage one another to prioritize rest in God and find solace in His presence within our Christian community?

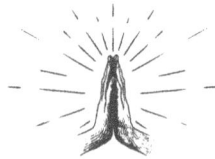

PRAYER

Heavenly Father, we thank you for the invitation to find rest in your presence. Help us to come to you with our burdens and worries, trusting in your provision and care. Teach us to take your yoke upon us and learn from you, finding strength and guidance for the journey. May we find true rest for our souls as we abide in you. In Jesus' name, we pray, Amen.

WEEK 34:

CULTIVATING JOY

PHILIPPIANS 4:4 (NIV)

"Rejoice in the Lord always. I will say it again: Rejoice!"

DEVOTION

In Philippians 4:4, the apostle Paul exhorts believers to rejoice in the Lord always—a command that transcends circumstances and invites us into a lifestyle of joy. Joy is not merely a fleeting emotion dependent on our external circumstances, but a deep-seated disposition of the heart rooted in our relationship with God.

Cultivating joy involves a deliberate choice—a conscious decision to focus on the goodness and faithfulness of God rather than on the challenges and trials of life. It means finding reasons to rejoice in every situation, knowing that our ultimate source of joy is found in the unchanging character of God and the salvation we have in Christ.

Moreover, joy is not dependent on our own strength or efforts but is a fruit of the Spirit—a gift freely given to us by God. As we abide in Him and allow His Spirit to work within us, joy naturally flows from our relationship with Him. It is a manifestation of the inner transformation that takes place when we surrender our lives to Christ and allow His love to fill us to overflowing.

Choosing joy is not always easy, especially when faced with adversity or suffering. However, as we fix our eyes on Jesus and trust in His promises, our perspective shifts, and we are able to rejoice even in the midst of trials. Joy becomes a source of strength and resilience, enabling us to persevere with hope and confidence in God's faithfulness.

DISCUSSION QUESTIONS

How does Philippians 4:4 challenge our understanding of joy and rejoicing?

Reflecting on your own life, what are some obstacles that hinder your ability to cultivate joy?

In what ways can we practice rejoicing in the Lord always, regardless of our circumstances?

Share about a time when you experienced the transformative power of joy in the midst of difficulty.

How can we encourage one another to cultivate a spirit of joy within our Christian community?

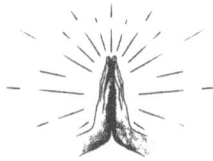

PRAYER

Heavenly Father, we thank you for the gift of joy that comes from knowing you and abiding in your love. Help us to rejoice in you always, regardless of our circumstances. May our hearts overflow with gratitude and praise as we fix our eyes on your goodness and faithfulness. Fill us afresh with your Spirit, that we may bear fruit of joy in every season of life. In Jesus' name, we pray, Amen.

GUARDING OUR THOUGHTS

PHILIPPIANS 4:8 (NIV)

"Finally, brothers and sisters, whatever is true, whatever is noble, whatever is right, whatever is pure, whatever is lovely, whatever is admirable—if anything is excellent or praiseworthy—think about such things."

DEVOTION

Philippians 4:8 provides a powerful exhortation to guard our thoughts and focus on things that are true, noble, right, pure, lovely, admirable, excellent, and praiseworthy. Our thoughts have a profound impact on our attitudes, emotions, and behaviors, shaping the trajectory of our lives. Therefore, it is crucial to be intentional about what we allow to occupy our minds.

In a world inundated with negativity, cynicism, and impurity, it can be challenging to maintain a mindset of excellence. However, as followers of Christ, we are called to a higher standard—a standard that reflects the character and values of God Himself. By aligning our thoughts with the qualities outlined in Philippians 4:8, we set ourselves apart from the patterns of the world and cultivate a mindset that honors God.

Guarding our thoughts involves discernment and discipline. It requires us to be vigilant in monitoring the influences that shape our thinking, whether through media, relationships, or our own internal dialogue. Instead of dwelling on negative or harmful thoughts, we intentionally redirect our focus toward things that are edifying, uplifting, and life-giving.

Moreover, the call to guard our thoughts extends beyond mere mental discipline—it is also a spiritual practice that invites God's presence and guidance into our lives. As we fix our minds on things that are true, noble, and praiseworthy, we create space for the Holy Spirit to work within us, transforming our hearts and renewing our minds according to God's truth.

DISCUSSION QUESTIONS

How does Philippians 4:8 challenge us to guard our thoughts and focus on things of excellence?

Reflecting on your own life, what are some common sources of negative or harmful thoughts that you encounter?

In what ways can we actively cultivate a mindset of excellence in our daily lives?

Share about a time when intentionally focusing on positive and uplifting thoughts impacted your attitude or perspective.

How can we support and encourage one another in the practice of guarding our thoughts within our Christian community?

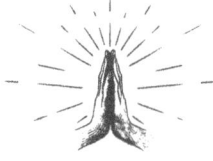

PRAYER

Heavenly Father, we thank you for the guidance of your Word in shaping our thoughts and attitudes. Help us to guard our minds diligently, focusing on things that are true, noble, and praiseworthy. May our thoughts reflect your character and values, bringing honor to your name. Fill us with your Spirit, that we may cultivate a mindset of excellence and be transformed by the renewing of our minds. In Jesus' name, we pray, Amen.

WEEK 36:

SEEKING MENTAL AND EMOTIONAL HEALING

JAMES 5:16 (NIV)

"Therefore confess your sins to each other and pray for each other so that you may be healed. The prayer of a righteous person is powerful and effective."

DEVOTION

In James 5:16, believers are encouraged to seek healing through prayer and mutual confession. This verse emphasizes the importance of spiritual and emotional healing, acknowledging the interconnectedness of our physical, mental, and spiritual well-being. As we come before God in prayer, confessing our sins and lifting up one another's needs, we open ourselves to His transformative power and restoration.

Seeking healing is a multifaceted journey that encompasses various aspects of our lives. It involves acknowledging our brokenness and need for God's intervention, as well as actively participating in the process of restoration through prayer, faith, and obedience to God's Word.

The prayer of a righteous person is powerful and effective—not because of our own righteousness, but because of the righteousness of Christ imputed to us through faith. When we approach God in humility and faith, trusting in His goodness and sovereignty, we unleash the power of prayer to bring about healing and wholeness in our lives and the lives of others.

Moreover, seeking healing is not merely about physical ailments or outward symptoms; it is also about inner transformation and spiritual renewal. As we confess our sins and submit to God's healing work in our hearts, He brings about healing and restoration on a deep, soul-level, freeing us from bondage and equipping us to live lives of purpose and fulfillment.

DISCUSSION QUESTIONS

How does James 5:16 challenge our understanding of healing and the role of prayer in the process?

Reflecting on your own experiences, in what areas of your life do you need healing—physically, emotionally, spiritually?

What barriers or misconceptions might hinder us from seeking healing through prayer and mutual confession?

Share about a time when you witnessed the power of prayer to bring about healing or restoration.

How can we cultivate a culture of prayer and mutual support within our Christian community to facilitate healing and spiritual growth?

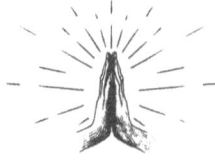

PRAYER

Heavenly Father, we thank you for the promise of healing and restoration through prayer and confession. Help us to come before you with humble and contrite hearts, acknowledging our need for healing and trusting in your power to bring about transformation. May we be faithful to pray for one another, lifting up each other's needs and believing in your faithfulness to answer according to your will. In Jesus' name, we pray, Amen.

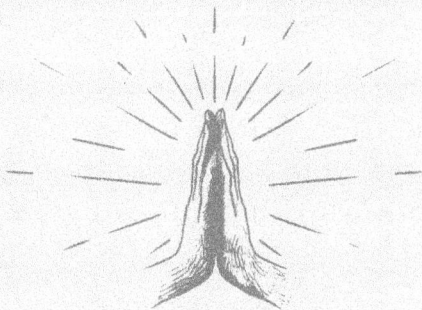

FINANCIAL HEALTH

WEEK 37:

STEWARDSHIP

PSALM 24:1 (NIV)

"The earth is the Lord's, and everything in it,
the world, and all who live in it."

DEVOTION

Psalm 24:1 reminds us of the fundamental truth that God is the Creator and Owner of all things. As stewards of God's creation, we are called to recognize and honor His sovereignty by responsibly managing the resources He has entrusted to us. Stewardship encompasses every aspect of our lives— our time, talents, finances, and relationships—and it is a reflection of our love for God and our commitment to His purposes.

Understanding that everything belongs to God transforms our perspective on possessions and wealth. Rather than viewing them as solely ours to use for our own pleasure or gain, we recognize them as gifts from God to be used wisely and generously for His glory and the betterment of others. Stewardship involves acknowledging God's ownership, seeking His guidance in decision-making, and faithfully stewarding His resources according to His will.

Moreover, stewardship extends beyond material possessions to include our time and talents. How we invest our time and utilize our gifts reflects our priorities and values. As stewards, we are called to be intentional in using our time and talents for Kingdom purposes, serving others, and advancing God's work in the world.

DISCUSSION QUESTIONS

How does Psalm 24:1 challenge our understanding of ownership and stewardship?

Reflecting on your own life, what are some areas in which you struggle to be a faithful steward of God's resources?

In what ways can we practice stewardship in our daily lives, including our finances, time, talents, and relationships?

Share about a time when practicing stewardship led to a deeper sense of obedience and alignment with God's purposes.

How can we encourage one another to be faithful stewards within our Christian community?

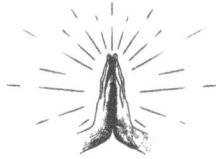

PRAYER

Heavenly Father, we thank you for the privilege of being entrusted with your resources. Help us to be faithful stewards of all that you have given us, recognizing your ownership and seeking to honor you in our use of time, talents, and finances. Grant us wisdom and discernment to manage your resources wisely and generously for your Kingdom purposes. May our stewardship bring glory to your name and bear fruit that lasts for eternity. In Jesus' name, we pray, Amen.

WEEK 38:

GENEROSITY

2 CORINTHIANS 9:7 (NIV)

"Each of you should give what you have decided in your heart to give, not reluctantly or under compulsion, for God loves a cheerful giver."

DEVOTION

In 2 Corinthians 9:7, Paul encourages believers to embrace a spirit of generosity in their giving. Generosity is more than just an act of charity; it is a reflection of the generous nature of our Heavenly Father and an expression of our gratitude for His blessings in our lives.

True generosity flows from the heart—a voluntary response to God's grace and provision. It is not motivated by obligation or compulsion but by a joyful desire to share the blessings we have received with others. When we give with a cheerful heart, we align ourselves with God's purposes and experience the joy of participating in His work of blessing and provision.

Furthermore, generosity is not limited to financial giving; it encompasses all aspects of our lives. We can be generous with our time, talents, resources, and love, using whatever God has entrusted to us to bless others and advance His Kingdom. As we cultivate a spirit of generosity, we become channels of God's grace, bringing light and hope to those in need.

DISCUSSION QUESTIONS

How does 2 Corinthians 9:7 challenge our understanding of generosity and giving?

Reflecting on your own life, what are some blessings you have received that you can share with others?

In what ways can we practice generosity in our daily lives, beyond financial giving?

Share about a time when you experienced the joy of giving and blessing others.

How can we cultivate a culture of generosity within our Christian community?

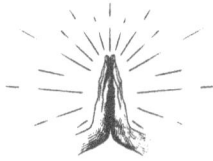

PRAYER

Heavenly Father, we thank you for your abundant blessings in our lives. Help us to be cheerful givers, freely sharing the blessings we have received with others. May our generosity reflect your love and grace, bringing hope and joy to those in need. Give us hearts that are open and willing to give, not out of compulsion, but out of a desire to honor you and bless others. In Jesus' name, we pray, Amen.

WEEK 39:

CONTENTMENT

PHILIPPIANS 4:11-12 (NIV)

"I have learned to be content whatever the circumstances. I know what it is to be in need, and I know what it is to have plenty. I have learned the secret of being content in any and every situation, whether well fed or hungry, whether living in plenty or in want."

DEVOTION

In Philippians 4:11-12, the apostle Paul shares his secret to contentment—a mindset that remains steadfast regardless of life's circumstances. Contentment is not dependent on external factors such as wealth, status, or possessions, but on an inner attitude of gratitude and trust in God's provision.

Paul's words remind us that contentment is a learned behavior—a discipline cultivated over time through experience and reliance on God's faithfulness. It is a state of heart and mind that transcends our circumstances, enabling us to find peace and satisfaction in every season of life.

Contentment does not mean that we become complacent or indifferent to our circumstances; rather, it empowers us to navigate life's ups and downs with grace and resilience. Whether we are experiencing abundance or scarcity, joy or sorrow, contentment enables us to remain anchored in God's unchanging love and provision.

Moreover, contentment frees us from the pursuit of worldly wealth and possessions, allowing us to prioritize the things that truly matter—our relationship with God, our loved ones, and the advancement of His Kingdom. It liberates us from the grip of materialism and consumerism, leading to a simpler, more meaningful way of life.

DISCUSSION QUESTIONS

How does Philippians 4:11-12 challenge our understanding of contentment and satisfaction?

Reflecting on your own life, what are some factors that hinder your ability to be content in all circumstances?

In what ways can we practice contentment in our daily lives, regardless of our circumstances?

Share about a time when you experienced contentment despite facing challenges or difficulties.

How can we encourage one another to cultivate a spirit of contentment within our Christian community?

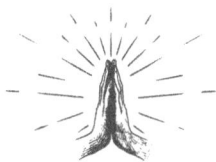

PRAYER

Heavenly Father, we thank you for your provision and faithfulness in every season of life. Help us to cultivate a spirit of contentment, finding satisfaction in your love and provision rather than in worldly wealth or possessions. Teach us to trust in your timing and sovereignty, knowing that you are always working for our good. May our hearts overflow with gratitude and peace as we rest in your unfailing love. In Jesus' name, we pray, Amen.

WEEK 40:

AVOIDING DEBT

PROVERBS 22:7 (NIV)

"The rich rule over the poor, and the borrower is slave to the lender."

DEVOTION

Proverbs 22:7 offers a sobering reminder of the dangers of debt and the potential consequences of financial irresponsibility. Debt has a way of enslaving us, limiting our freedom and autonomy, and often leading to stress, anxiety, and relational strain. As followers of Christ, we are called to exercise wisdom and stewardship in all areas of our lives, including our finances.

Avoiding debt is not merely a matter of financial prudence but also a reflection of our trust in God's provision and sovereignty. When we live within our means and avoid the allure of easy credit, we demonstrate our reliance on God as our ultimate provider and sustainer. We acknowledge that true security and fulfillment are found in Him, not in material possessions or worldly wealth.

Moreover, living debt-free enables us to be more generous and compassionate toward others, as we are freed from the burden of debt repayment and can more readily respond to the needs of those around us. It allows us to invest in

Kingdom purposes and advance God's work in the world, rather than being consumed by the pursuit of personal gain.

DISCUSSION QUESTIONS

How does Proverbs 22:7 challenge our understanding of debt and financial stewardship?

Reflecting on your own financial habits, what are some factors that can lead to indebtedness?

In what ways can we practice financial wisdom and avoid debt in our daily lives?

Share about a time when you experienced the consequences of debt or witnessed its impact on others.

How can we support and encourage one another in pursuing financial freedom within our Christian community?

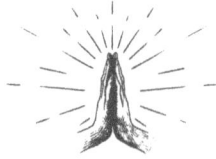

PRAYER

Heavenly Father, we thank you for your provision and guidance in all areas of our lives, including our finances. Help us to be wise stewards of the resources you have entrusted to us, avoiding the trap of debt and living within our means. Give us discernment to make sound financial decisions and the discipline to resist the lure of easy credit. May our lives reflect your wisdom and generosity, bringing glory to your name. In Jesus' name, we pray, Amen.

WEEK 41:

PLANNING AND BUDGETING

PROVERBS 21:5 (NIV)

*"The plans of the diligent lead to profit as
surely as haste leads to poverty."*

DEVOTION

Proverbs 21:5 emphasizes the importance of diligent planning and wise stewardship in managing our finances. Planning and budgeting are essential components of responsible financial management, enabling us to make informed decisions, prioritize our spending, and achieve our long-term goals.

Financial planning begins with setting clear objectives and identifying our sources of income and expenses. By creating a budget that aligns with our priorities and values, we gain greater control over our finances and are better equipped to handle unexpected expenses or financial challenges that may arise.

Moreover, planning and budgeting foster discipline and self-control, helping us to avoid impulsive spending and unnecessary debt. When we steward our resources wisely and live within our means, we honor God with our finances and position ourselves for long-term financial stability and success.

As Christians, our approach to planning and budgeting should be guided by biblical principles, such as generosity, stewardship, and trust in God's provision. We recognize that our financial resources ultimately belong to God, and we seek His wisdom and guidance in managing them effectively for His glory and purposes.

DISCUSSION QUESTIONS

How does Proverbs 21:5 challenge our understanding of planning and budgeting?

Reflecting on your own financial habits, what are some areas where you could improve your planning and budgeting?

In what ways can we incorporate biblical principles into our approach to financial planning and budgeting?

Share about a time when diligent planning and budgeting led to positive financial outcomes in your life.

How can we support and encourage one another in developing and maintaining healthy financial habits within our Christian community?

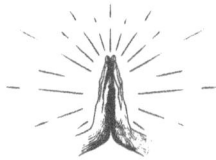

PRAYER

Heavenly Father, we thank you for the wisdom and guidance you provide us in managing our finances. Help us to be diligent in our planning and budgeting, seeking your guidance in all our financial decisions. Give us wisdom to set priorities, discipline to stick to our budgets, and faith to trust in your provision. May our financial stewardship honor you and reflect your goodness to others. In Jesus' name, we pray, Amen.

WEEK 42:

HARD WORK AND DILIGENCE

PROVERBS 10:4 (NIV)

"Lazy hands make for poverty, but diligent hands bring wealth."

DEVOTION

Proverbs 10:4 underscores the importance of hard work and diligence in achieving success and prosperity. Diligence involves persistent effort, perseverance, and a commitment to excellence in all that we do. It is a virtue that honors God and positions us for opportunities and blessings.

Hard work is a biblical principle woven throughout Scripture, reflecting God's design for human productivity and stewardship. From the creation mandate in Genesis to the exhortations in the New Testament, Scripture consistently affirms the value of honest labor and the rewards that come from it.

Diligent hands bring wealth not only in terms of material prosperity but also in the form of personal growth, character development, and the ability to contribute positively to society. When we approach our work with diligence and integrity, we reflect the image of God and bear witness to His faithfulness and provision.

Moreover, diligence is not just about achieving worldly success; it is also about stewarding the gifts and talents God has given us for His purposes. Whether in our careers, relationships, or ministries, we are called to invest our time and energy wisely, using our abilities to glorify God and serve others.

DISCUSSION QUESTIONS

How does Proverbs 10:4 challenge our understanding of hard work and diligence?

Reflecting on your own work ethic, what are some areas where you could grow in diligence?

In what ways can we cultivate a spirit of diligence in our daily lives, both in our professional and personal pursuits?

Share about a time when your diligence led to success or positive outcomes.

How can we encourage one another to embrace a mindset of diligence and excellence within our Christian community?

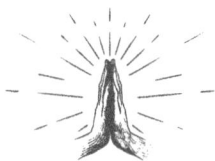

PRAYER

Heavenly Father, we thank you for the gift of work and the opportunity to steward the talents and abilities you have given us. Help us to approach our tasks with diligence and excellence, honoring you in all that we do. Grant us the strength and perseverance to work hard, knowing that our labor is not in vain when done for your glory. May our lives be a testimony to your faithfulness and provision. In Jesus' name, we pray, Amen.

WEEK 43:

SEEKING WISDOM

PROVERBS 16:16 (NIV)

*"How much better to get wisdom than gold,
to get insight rather than silver!"*

DEVOTION

Proverbs 16:16 presents a powerful comparison between the value of wisdom and material wealth. While riches may offer temporary comfort and security, true wisdom brings lasting benefits and eternal significance. Seeking wisdom is not merely a pursuit of knowledge but a quest for understanding, discernment, and insight into God's ways and purposes.

Wisdom is a precious gift from God, bestowed upon those who seek it with humility and sincerity. It enables us to navigate life's complexities with clarity and discernment, making wise decisions that honor God and benefit others. As we cultivate a heart of wisdom, we align ourselves with God's will and experience His guidance and provision in every aspect of our lives.

Moreover, wisdom is not confined to academic knowledge or intellectual prowess; it encompasses spiritual discernment and practical insight. It involves knowing how to apply God's truth to our daily circumstances and relationships, living in alignment with His principles and values.

As Christians, our pursuit of wisdom begins with the fear of the Lord—an awe and reverence for His holiness and authority. It is through our relationship with God and His Word that we find the source of true wisdom and understanding. As we seek His guidance in prayer and study His Word with an open heart, He imparts wisdom to us, enabling us to walk in His ways and fulfill His purposes.

DISCUSSION QUESTIONS

How does Proverbs 16:16 challenge our understanding of wisdom and its value?

Reflecting on your own life, what are some areas where you desire greater wisdom and understanding?

In what ways can we actively seek wisdom in our daily lives, both spiritually and practically?

Share about a time when seeking wisdom led to positive outcomes or spiritual growth in your life.

How can we encourage one another to prioritize the pursuit of wisdom within our Christian community?

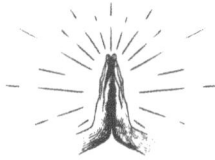

PRAYER

Heavenly Father, we thank you for the precious gift of wisdom that you offer to those who seek it. Grant us hearts that hunger and thirst for your wisdom, above all earthly riches and treasures. May we diligently seek understanding and discernment, knowing that true wisdom comes from you alone. Fill us with your Holy Spirit, that we may walk in wisdom and live according to your will. In Jesus' name, we pray, Amen.

HONESTY AND INTEGRITY

PROVERBS 11:1 (NIV)

"The Lord detests dishonest scales,
but accurate weights find favor with him."

DEVOTION

Proverbs 11:1 highlights the importance of honesty and integrity in our dealings with others. The imagery of "dishonest scales" refers to deceitful practices in business transactions, where individuals manipulate weights to deceive and exploit others. In contrast, "accurate weights" represent integrity and fairness, which find favor in the eyes of the Lord.

Honesty and integrity are foundational virtues that reflect our character and shape our interactions with others. They involve speaking truthfully, acting with sincerity, and upholding moral principles even when faced with temptation or pressure to compromise. As followers of Christ, we are called to be people of integrity, whose words and actions align with God's truth and righteousness.

Moreover, honesty and integrity are not merely external behaviors but spring from a heart that is transformed by

God's grace. When we walk in honesty and integrity, we honor God and bear witness to His character of truth and righteousness. Our integrity becomes a testimony to the world of the transformative power of the Gospel and the reality of God's presence in our lives.

DISCUSSION QUESTIONS

How does Proverbs 11:1 challenge our understanding of honesty and integrity?

Reflecting on your own life, what are some areas where honesty and integrity are tested?

In what ways can we cultivate a lifestyle of honesty and integrity in our daily interactions and relationships?

Share about a time when you witnessed the impact of honesty and integrity in your own life or the life of someone else.

How can we support and encourage one another to uphold honesty and integrity within our Christian community?

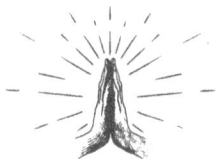

PRAYER

Heavenly Father, we thank you for your faithfulness and righteousness. Help us to walk in honesty and integrity, reflecting your character of truth and righteousness in all that we do. Guard our hearts from deceit and dishonesty, and empower us to speak truthfully and act with integrity in every circumstance. May our lives bring glory to your name and bear witness to your transforming power. In Jesus' name, we pray, Amen.

WEEK 45:
AVOIDING GREED

LUKE 12:15 (NIV)

"Then he said to them, 'Watch out! Be on your guard against all kinds of greed; life does not consist in an abundance of possessions.'"

DEVOTION

In Luke 12:15, Jesus warns His disciples against the dangers of greed, emphasizing that life's true value is not measured by the accumulation of possessions. Greed is a desire for more than what is needed, a relentless pursuit of wealth and material gain that often leads to discontentment, selfishness, and a neglect of spiritual priorities.

Greed is a subtle and insidious temptation that can easily entangle our hearts and minds if left unchecked. In a culture that often equates success and happiness with material wealth, it is easy to become consumed by the pursuit of possessions and financial security, losing sight of the things that truly matter—our relationship with God and our love for others.

Choosing contentment over greed requires a deliberate shift in perspective—a recognition that true fulfillment and joy are found in knowing and serving God, rather than in the abundance of earthly possessions. It involves cultivating a spirit of gratitude for what we have been given and trusting in God's provision for our needs.

Moreover, avoiding greed involves stewarding our resources wisely and generously, recognizing that everything we have ultimately belongs to God. As faithful stewards, we are called to use our resources to bless others, rather than hoarding them for our own gain. When we prioritize the needs of others and invest in Kingdom purposes, we experience the joy and satisfaction that comes from aligning our hearts with God's will.

DISCUSSION QUESTIONS

How does Luke 12:15 challenge our understanding of greed and its consequences?

Reflecting on your own life, what are some ways in which greed manifests itself in modern society?

In what ways can we cultivate a spirit of contentment and generosity in our daily lives?

Share about a time when you experienced the freedom and joy of choosing contentment over greed.

How can we support and encourage one another to resist the temptation of greed within our Christian community?

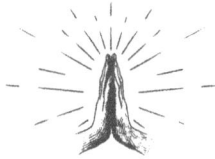

PRAYER

Heavenly Father, we confess our tendency to be swayed by the lure of greed and materialism. Help us to guard our hearts against the love of money and possessions, and to find our true satisfaction and security in you alone. Grant us the grace to cultivate a spirit of contentment, gratitude, and generosity, that we may reflect your character of love and selflessness in all that we do. In Jesus' name, we pray, Amen.

WEEK 46:
TRUSTING GOD FOR PROVISION

MATTHEW 6:25-34 (NIV)

"Therefore I tell you, do not worry about your life, what you will eat or drink; or about your body, what you will wear... Look at the birds of the air; they do not sow or reap or store away in barns, and yet your heavenly Father feeds them. Are you not much more valuable than they?... But seek first his kingdom and his righteousness, and all these things will be given to you as well."

DEVOTION

In Matthew 6:25-34, Jesus reassures His disciples that God is their faithful provider and urges them not to worry about their basic needs. He points to the birds of the air and the flowers of the field as examples of God's care and provision, highlighting the value of trusting in His sovereignty and goodness.

Trusting God for provision involves surrendering our worries and anxieties to Him and choosing to place our confidence in His faithfulness. It requires a shift in perspective—from a mindset of scarcity and self-reliance to one of abundance and dependence on God's grace. When we seek first God's Kingdom and righteousness, prioritizing His purposes above our own desires, He promises to meet all our needs according to His riches and glory.

Moreover, trusting God for provision is not passive; it is an active response of faith and obedience. It involves stewarding our resources wisely, being content with what we have, and sharing generously with others. As we step out in faith, God honors our obedience and provides for us in ways that exceed our expectations.

DISCUSSION QUESTIONS

How does Matthew 6:25-34 challenge our tendency to worry about our provision?

Reflecting on your own life, what are some areas where you struggle to trust God for provision?

In what ways can we cultivate a spirit of trust and dependence on God in our daily lives?

Share about a time when you experienced God's provision in a tangible way.

How can we support and encourage one another to trust God for provision within our Christian community?

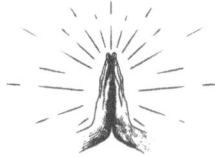

PRAYER

Heavenly Father, we thank you for your faithful provision and care for us. Help us to trust in your sovereignty and goodness, knowing that you are our loving Father who knows our needs and provides for us abundantly. Give us the faith to surrender our worries and anxieties to you, and to seek first your Kingdom and righteousness in all that we do. May our lives be a testimony to your faithfulness and grace. In Jesus' name, we pray, Amen.

WEEK 47:

INVESTING IN
ETERNAL TREASURES

MATTHEW 6:19-21 (NIV)

"Do not store up for yourselves treasures on earth, where moths and vermin destroy, and where thieves break in and steal. But store up for yourselves treasures in heaven, where moths and vermin do not destroy, and where thieves do not break in and steal. For where your treasure is, there your heart will be also."

DEVOTION

In Matthew 6:19-21, Jesus urges His disciples to prioritize eternal treasures over temporary earthly possessions. He warns against placing too much emphasis on accumulating wealth and material possessions, which are vulnerable to decay and loss. Instead, He encourages us to invest in treasures that have lasting value—treasures stored up in heaven, where they are secure and imperishable.

Investing in eternal treasures involves a shift in perspective—a recognition that true wealth and fulfillment are found in knowing and serving God, rather than in the accumulation of worldly goods. It requires a reordering of our priorities, aligning our hearts with the Kingdom of God and His purposes. As we invest our time, talents, and resources in Kingdom endeavors, we lay up treasures that will endure for eternity.

Moreover, investing in eternal treasures is a reflection of our faith and trust in God's promises. It involves stepping out in obedience, even when it requires sacrificial giving and self-denial. When we invest in Kingdom work—such as sharing the Gospel, serving others, and supporting ministries—we participate in God's redemptive plan and store up rewards that far surpass anything this world has to offer.

DISCUSSION QUESTIONS

How does Matthew 6:19-21 challenge our understanding of wealth and material possessions?

Reflecting on your own life, what are some ways you can invest in eternal treasures?

In what areas of your life do you struggle to prioritize eternal treasures over earthly possessions?

Share about a time when you witnessed the impact of investing in Kingdom work.

How can we encourage one another to invest in eternal treasures within our Christian community?

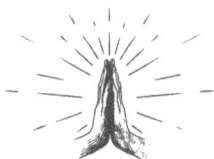

PRAYER

Heavenly Father, we thank you for the invitation to invest in eternal treasures and participate in your Kingdom work. Help us to cultivate hearts that are set on things above, rather than on earthly possessions. Give us wisdom to steward our resources faithfully and to invest in endeavors that advance your Kingdom and glorify your name. May our lives be a testimony to the surpassing value of knowing and serving you. In Jesus' name, we pray, Amen.

WEEK 48:

SEEKING GOD'S KINGDOM FIRST

LUKE 12:31 (NIV)

"But seek his kingdom, and these things will be given to you as well."

DEVOTION

In the midst of life's uncertainties and worries, Jesus offers a simple yet profound directive in Luke 12:31: "But seek his kingdom, and these things will be given to you as well." This statement encapsulates the essence of a life transformed by the pursuit of God's kingdom.

To seek God's kingdom first is to prioritize His reign and rule in our lives above all else. It involves aligning our desires, ambitions, and actions with the principles and values of His kingdom. Instead of being consumed by the pursuit of material wealth, status, or success, we are called to pursue the things that matter most to God—righteousness, love, mercy, and justice.

Seeking God's kingdom requires a radical shift in perspective. It means recognizing that true fulfillment and abundance are found not in the accumulation of worldly possessions but in the presence and purposes of God. As we seek

His kingdom above all else, we discover a deeper sense of purpose and meaning in our lives, rooted in our relationship with Him.

Jesus assures us that when we prioritize seeking His kingdom, our needs will be met. This doesn't mean that we will be exempt from challenges or hardships, but it means that God will provide for us according to His abundant grace and generosity. As we entrust our lives to Him and seek His kingdom first, we can rest in the assurance that He is faithful to meet our needs according to His perfect will.

Furthermore, seeking God's kingdom is not just an individual pursuit but a collective endeavor. As members of the body of Christ, we are called to partner with God in advancing His kingdom here on earth. This involves sharing the message of salvation, demonstrating His love and compassion to others, and working for justice and reconciliation in our communities.

As we embark on the journey of seeking God's kingdom first, may we be transformed by His grace and empowered by His Spirit. May our lives bear witness to the transformative power of living in alignment with His kingdom values, bringing glory to His name and drawing others into the abundant life found in Him.

DISCUSSION QUESTIONS

What does it mean to seek God's kingdom in your everyday life? How does this influence your priorities and decisions?

Can you share a personal experience of how prioritizing God's kingdom has impacted your perspective on material possessions and worldly success?

In what ways do you see the values of God's kingdom diverging from the values of the world? How can we navigate this contrast as followers of Christ?

How can we encourage and support one another in the pursuit of God's kingdom within our families, churches, and communities?

What practical steps can we take to prioritize seeking God's kingdom first in our daily routines and interactions with others?

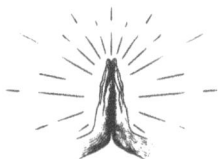

PRAYER

Heavenly Father, we thank you for the invitation to seek your kingdom first and prioritize your righteousness in our lives. Help us to surrender our desires and ambitions to your will, and to align our hearts with your Kingdom purposes. Give us the strength and perseverance to pursue righteousness and obedience, trusting in your provision and guidance. May our lives bring glory to your name as we seek first your kingdom. In Jesus' name, we pray, Amen.

CONCLUSION
(THE WRAP UP)

As we conclude this 48-week journey through the principles of Christian holistic health, we are reminded of the profound interconnectedness of our spiritual, physical, mental, and financial well-being. Over the past year, we have explored the timeless wisdom of Scripture and practical insights for nurturing each aspect of our lives in alignment with God's design.

Throughout this devotional, we have learned that true health and wholeness come from embracing God's holistic vision for our lives—a vision that encompasses every dimension of our being. We have discovered that spiritual health is foundational, as it shapes our perspective, priorities, and purpose. Through prayer, Scripture study, worship, and fellowship, we deepen our relationship with God and align our lives with His Kingdom purposes.

We have also explored the importance of physical health, recognizing our bodies as temples of the Holy Spirit. By nourishing our bodies with healthy food, engaging in regular exercise, prioritizing rest, and avoiding harmful habits, we honor God and steward our physical well-being for His glory.

Mental health has been another focal point of our journey, as we've learned to care for our minds and emotions. By renewing our minds with God's Word, managing stress, seeking support when needed, and practicing self-care, we cultivate mental resilience and emotional balance in the midst of life's challenges.

Finally, we have examined the significance of financial health, understanding that stewardship is an expression of our trust in God's provision. By living within our means, avoiding debt, practicing generosity, and using our resources to advance God's Kingdom purposes, we align our finances with His priorities and experience the freedom that comes from trusting in His provision.

As we conclude this devotional journey, may we continue to pursue holistic health in every area of our lives, knowing that true flourishing comes from surrendering all aspects of our being to God's loving care. May we walk in obedience to His Word, seeking His Kingdom first and trusting in His promise to provide for all our needs. And may our lives be a testimony to the transformative power of God's grace, as we strive to honor Him with our whole selves—spiritually, physically, mentally, and financially. Amen.